Workbook for Hartman's Medical Assisting

The Basics

by Hartman Publishing, Inc.

hartmanonline.com

Hartman

Credits

Managing Editor
Susan Alvare Hedman

Developmental Editor
Kristin Calderon

Cover Designer
Kirsten Browne

Production
Tracy Kopsachilis

Proofreaders
Juliann Barbato
Danielle Lescure
Kathi Minton
Charity Smith
Megan Whelan

Copyright Information

1313 Iron Avenue SW
Albuquerque, New Mexico 87102
(505) 291-1274
web: hartmanonline.com
email: orders@hartmanonline.com
Twitter: @HartmanPub

ISBN 978-1-60425-149-4

PRINTED IN THE USA

Notice to Readers

Though the guidelines and procedures contained in this text are based on consultations with healthcare professionals, they should not be considered absolute recommendations. The instructor and readers should follow employer, local, state, and federal guidelines concerning healthcare practices. These guidelines change, and it is the reader's responsibility to be aware of these changes and of the policies and procedures of their healthcare facility.

The publisher, author, editors, and reviewers cannot accept any responsibility for errors or omissions or for any consequences from application of the information in this book and make no warranty, express or implied, with respect to the contents of the book. The publisher does not warrant or guarantee any of the products described herein or perform any analysis in connection with any of the product information contained herein.

Gender Usage

This workbook uses gender pronouns interchangeably to denote healthcare team members and patients.

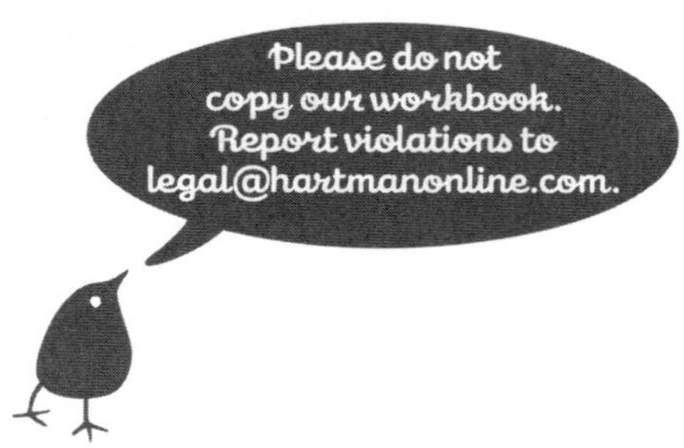

Table of Contents

Preface v

Lesson Plans

1 The Role of the Medical Assistant 1

2 Legal and Ethical Issues 5

3 Communication and Diversity 13

4 Psychology and Human Needs and Development 21

5 Infection Prevention and Control 27

6 Safety, Emergency Care, and Disaster Preparation 35

7 Patient Scheduling, Reception, and Related Communication 41

8 Medical Record Management 47

9 Medical Insurance and Coding 51

10 Billing, Collections, and Accounting 57

11 Office Equipment and Supplies 61

12 Introduction to Medical Terminology and Body Systems 65

13 Basic Clinical Skills 69

14 The Integumentary System and Related Care 83

15 The Musculoskeletal System and Related Care 87

16 The Nervous System and Sense Organs and Related Care 95

17 The Circulatory System and Related Care 103

18 The Respiratory System and Related Care 109

19 The Urinary System and Related Care 117

20 The Gastrointestinal System and Related Care 123

21 The Endocrine System and Related Care 131

22 The Reproductive System and Related Care 137

23 The Immune and Lymphatic Systems and Related Care 145

24 Phlebotomy and Common Blood Tests 151

25 Electrocardiograms (EKGs) and Related Tests 159

26 Pharmacology and Medication Administration 167

Procedure Checklists 175

Practice Exam 213

Preface

Welcome to the *Workbook for Hartman's Medical Assisting: The Basics*! This workbook is designed to help you review what you have learned from reading your textbook. For this reason, the workbook is organized around learning objectives, just like the textbook and your instructor's teaching material.

These learning objectives work as a built-in study guide. After completing the exercises for each learning objective in the workbook, ask yourself if you can *do* what that learning objective describes.

If you can, move on to the next learning objective. If you cannot, go back to the textbook, reread that learning objective, and try again.

We have provided procedure checklists close to the end of the workbook. There is also a practice test for the certification exam. The answers to the workbook exercises are in your instructor's teaching guide.

Happy learning!

Name: ______________________

1
The Role of the Medical Assistant

1. Explain the medical assistant's role

Multiple Choice

Circle the letter of the answer that best completes the statement or answers the question.

1. One common role of the MA is acting as a
   (A) Financial manager
   (B) Diagnostician
   (C) Patient counselor
   (D) Patient navigator

2. What type of care is given with an emphasis on staying healthy and avoiding serious injury?
   (A) Inpatient care
   (B) Preventive care
   (C) Ambulatory care
   (D) Emergency care

3. Front-office work for an MA may include which of the following?
   (A) Measuring and recording patient vital signs
   (B) Assisting the provider with minor surgical procedures
   (C) Taking a patient's medical history
   (D) Greeting and registering patients

4. What is the term for getting approval from a patient's health insurance company before a procedure is done?
   (A) Scheduling
   (B) Preauthorization
   (C) Practice management
   (D) Claim submission

5. Laboratory testing performed at a patient's side is known as
   (A) Acute care
   (B) Phlebotomy
   (C) Point-of-care testing
   (D) Direct care

6. Medical assistants
   (A) Sterilize equipment and supplies
   (B) Perform minor surgical procedures
   (C) Do not have any supervision
   (D) Share new diagnoses with patients

7. Collecting blood specimens from a vein or by skin puncture is called
   (A) Point-of-care testing
   (B) Diagnostic testing
   (C) Specimen processing
   (D) Phlebotomy

8. Under whose direction may an MA provide patient education?
   (A) The healthcare provider's
   (B) The patient's
   (C) The office manager's
   (D) The facility administrator's

Matching

For each of the following terms, write the letter of the correct definition. Use each letter only once.

9. ____ Patient navigator
10. ____ Coding
11. ____ Administrative
12. ____ Ambulatory care
13. ____ Preauthorization
14. ____ Clinical

(A) Related to the business and customer service operations of a medical office or other healthcare facility

(B) Related directly to patient care

(C) The role of facilitating a patient's health care and progress through the healthcare system

(D) An established way to document medical care provided

(E) Care given without the patient being admitted to a hospital

(F) The process of receiving approval from a patient's health insurance provider for procedures

2. Describe healthcare settings where medical assistants work

True or False

Mark each statement with either a T *for true or an* F *for false.*

1. T MAs may work in inpatient, outpatient, or home care settings.
2. T Most MAs work in outpatient healthcare settings.
3. F MAs have no role in care provided in a telehealth encounter.
4. F Geriatric medicine specialists provide care to patients 80 years of age and older.
5. T Internal medicine specialists provide preventive care, diagnosis, treatment, and management of conditions to adults of all ages.

3. Identify members of the healthcare team

Multiple Choice

1. This team member is not a physician but can perform many of the tasks of the physician, including prescribing medications:
   (A) Doctor of osteopathy
   (B) Registered nurse
   (C) Nurse practitioner
   (D) Patient care technician
2. This team member diagnoses and treats patients and usually supervises and directs the MA's work:
   (A) Registered nurse
   (B) Physician
   (C) Licensed practical nurse
   (D) Patient care technician
3. This team member can perform many of the clinical functions of the MA, but is not trained to give medications or perform administrative tasks:
   (A) Patient care technician
   (B) Phlebotomist
   (C) Administrative assistant
   (D) Licensed practical nurse

Short Answer

4. List and describe the two types of healthcare providers often called mid-level providers. Include the education they must have and the duties they are usually allowed to perform.

4. Understand delegation and scope of practice

True or False

1. T Triage is an example of a task that cannot be delegated to an MA.

Name: Rebeca

2. T A facility or office chain of command outlines who is accountable to whom and who reports to whom.
3. F There is a uniform scope of practice for MAs nationally.
4. T In general, tasks that require decision-making based on specific medical knowledge may not be delegated to an MA.
5. T If a state does not have laws about allowable tasks for MAs, the scope of practice is guided by the facility where the MA works.

5. Define professionalism and list examples of professional behavior

Multiple Choice

1. This characteristic involves making good judgments and maintaining confidentiality.
   (A) Dedication
   (B) Personability
   (C) Discretion
   (D) Honesty
2. Which of the following describes how an MA's fingernails should be kept?
   (A) Natural nails or artificial nails, trimmed short and kept clean
   (B) Short, clean natural nails and no chipped nail polish
   (C) Short, clean natural nails with wraps rather than polish
   (D) Short, clean natural nails with no polish or wraps
3. How should long hair be styled?
   (A) In a single braid down the back
   (B) With a part in the middle
   (C) Combed or brushed and pulled back in a ponytail or bun
   (D) Combed or brushed and covered with a hairnet

6. Describe the certification process

Short Answer

1. List two common requirements for MA certification.

____
____
____
____
____

2. List three benefits of being certified as an MA.

____
____
____
____
____
____
____
____
____
____

3. What are additional certifications an MA may choose to earn?

____
____
____
____

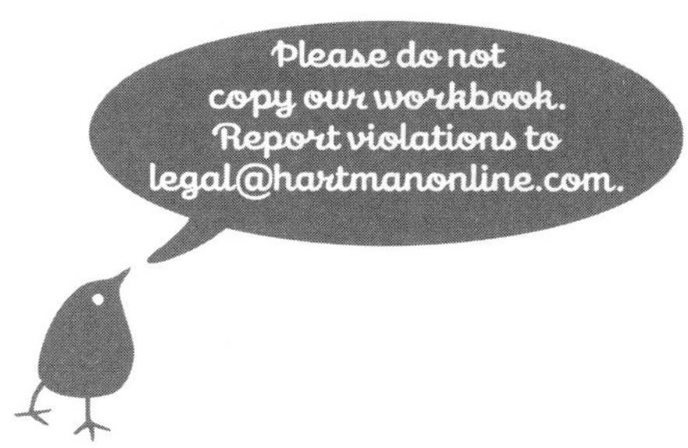

Name: ___________________________

2

Legal and Ethical Issues

1. Define the terms *law* and *ethics* and list examples of legal and ethical behavior

Short Answer

For each of the following examples, decide whether the issue is a legal issue or an ethical issue. Write L *for legal or* E *for ethical.*

1. _____ When Maria is at home with her husband she makes fun of the way one of the patients she sees speaks English.
2. _____ Dennis takes a book from a patient's purse while she is using the bathroom and gives it to a friend.
3. _____ Imani is 10 minutes late coming in for work on Monday. Her supervisor does not notice and Imani does not tell her.
4. _____ Rachel is excited to see that a well-known musician is a patient at the facility where she works. She opens his record and takes a photo to show her friends.

Read each of the following scenarios and answer the questions.

5. Sarah, an MA, is out shopping with her friends. One of them asks her if she likes her job, and she responds enthusiastically. She then tells them that one patient she saw that week, Mrs. Daly, has Alzheimer's disease and has to be reminded of her name often, as she is apt to forget it.

Did Sarah behave in a legal and ethical manner? Why or why not?

____

____

____

____

____

6. Caroyl works as an MA at a pediatrician's office. The mother of a patient who has been through a difficult illness pulls her aside after an appointment. She says that she really appreciates how kind Caroyl has been during these hard times. She gives her a wrapped present and says it is for all she has done for their family. Caroyl initially refuses, but after the mother insists, she takes it from her, thanking her.

Did Caroyl behave in a legal and ethical manner? Why or why not?

____

____

____

____

____

7. Mark, an MA, has been working at a geriatrics practice for almost a year. One patient is always accompanied by her daughter, Susan. During the course of conversation, Susan asks Mark to come have a drink with her so they can talk about her mother's care in a more relaxed environment. Mark tells her that he can go out for a short while after work that day. They arrange to meet.

Did Mark behave in a legal and ethical manner? Why or why not?

____

____

Name: ______________________

____

____

____

2. Explain patients' rights and why they are important

Multiple Choice

Read each of the following scenarios. Decide which of the patients' rights is being violated in each, and circle the correct letter.

1. Mrs. Perkins is a patient who is hearing impaired. She has hearing aids, but came to her appointment without them. Ethan, a medical assistant, is very frustrated as she struggles to hear him. As he leaves the exam room where Mrs. Perkins is waiting he sees the provider in the hallway walking another patient out. Ethan says, "Good luck talking to Mrs. Perkins today. She's deaf as a door." Which of the patients' rights is being violated?
   (A) The right to help with billing claims
   (B) The right to a clean and safe environment
   (C) The right to involvement in care
   (D) The right to protection of privacy

2. Mr. Gallerano has cancer and is undergoing chemotherapy. Kayla is an MA assigned to give him an injection to help with nausea. Kayla does not double-check the medication before injecting it. Only afterward does she realize she has given him the wrong drug. She knows the medication Mr. Gallerano accidentally received will not harm him. Because she is afraid of getting in trouble, she disposes of the syringe and documents that Mr. Gallerano received the correct drug. Which of the patients' rights is being violated?
   (A) The right to help with billing claims
   (B) The right to a clean and safe environment
   (C) The right to involvement in care
   (D) The right to protection of privacy

3. Ms. Mayes comes to the office with a deep cut from a knife that slipped while she was preparing dinner. Dr. Gonzales sees that she will need stitches and asks Rick to prepare the procedure room. The suture kit Rick takes from the supply room seems like someone may have started to open it before. He is not sure it is sterile, but he is in a hurry, so he uses it anyway. Which of the patients' rights is being violated?
   (A) The right to help with billing claims
   (B) The right to a clean and safe environment
   (C) The right to involvement in care
   (D) The right to protection of privacy

4. Jasmine is a medical assistant at a pediatric oncology office. Every night when she goes home, she tells her family touching stories about the patients with whom she works. Which of the patients' rights is being violated?
   (A) The right to help with billing claims
   (B) The right to a clean and safe environment
   (C) The right to involvement in care
   (D) The right to protection of privacy

5. Sofia, a medical assistant with an agency that does home visits for a life insurance company, is running behind with her work for the day. Both Mr. and Mrs. Bjerk are applying for coverage. Mrs. Bjerk is late coming home from an errand and Sofia has finished taking Mr. Bjerk's vital signs, reviewing his history, and getting his blood drawn. When Mrs. Bjerk arrives, Sofia decides to just take her blood and make up the rest to save time. After all, Mrs. Bjerk seems healthy and already filled out a history form online. Which of the patients' rights is being violated?
   (A) The right to high-quality care
   (B) The right to a clean and safe environment
   (C) The right to help with billing claims
   (D) The right to protection of privacy

6. Malik is a medical assistant at a family practice. A family of five comes in for flu shots. Malik gives shots to the parents and two of the children. The oldest child is terrified of shots. Malik says, "You're the oldest kid in your family. Didn't you see your baby brother take his shot? Are you a bigger baby than he is?" Which of the patients' rights is being violated?
   (A) The right to high-quality care
   (B) The right to help with follow-up care
   (C) The right to help with billing claims
   (D) The right to protection of privacy

7. Ms. Land, an elderly patient, is experiencing confusion. Her doctor thinks she may have a urinary tract infection and asks Theresa, a medical assistant, to get a urine specimen. Ms. Land says she does not want to give a specimen. Theresa tells her she is being very naughty and will not be allowed to leave the office until she provides the specimen. Which of the patients' rights is being violated?
   (A) The right to help with billing claims
   (B) The right to help with follow-up care
   (C) The right to involvement in care
   (D) The right to protection of privacy

8. Angie, a medical assistant, is supposed to go over the expected costs of an outpatient procedure with Mr. Diewald before the procedure is performed. It is a busy day, however, and so she just hands him several sheets of paper describing the procedure and related costs. He signs saying he received the information. After the procedure Mr. Diewald receives his bill and is surprised by the amount he owes. He calls the office and tells Angie he has just been laid off and does not have the money to pay his bill. Angie says, "I'm sorry, Mr. Diewald, but you should have known the cost beforehand. It was on your paperwork. You're just going to have to figure it out." Which of the patients' rights is being violated?
   (A) The right to high-quality care
   (B) The right to help with follow-up care
   (C) The right to help with billing claims
   (D) The right to protection of privacy

3. Explain HIPAA and discuss ways to protect patients' privacy

Multiple Choice

1. What is the purpose of the Health Insurance Portability and Accountability Act (HIPAA)?
   (A) To monitor quality of care in medical facilities
   (B) To protect and secure the privacy of health information
   (C) To reduce incidents of patient abuse
   (D) To provide health insurance for uninsured elderly people

2. What is included under protected health information (PHI)?
   (A) Patient's favorite food
   (B) Patient's favorite color
   (C) Patient's social security number
   (D) Patient's library card number

3. What is the correct response by a medical assistant if someone who is not directly involved with a patient's care asks for a patient's PHI?
   (A) Give them the information
   (B) Ask the patient if they may have the information
   (C) Ask them to ask the doctor
   (D) Tell them that the information is confidential and cannot be shared

4. Which of the following is one way to keep private health information confidential?
   (A) Making comments about patients on Twitter
   (B) Discussing patients' diagnoses with a coworker in a restaurant
   (C) Using confidential rooms for reporting on patients
   (D) Only discussing patients' conditions with trusted family members

5. The abbreviation for a law that was enacted as a part of the American Recovery and Reinvestment Act of 2009 to expand the protection and security of consumers' electronic health records (EHR) is called
   (A) HISEAL
   (B) HITECH
   (C) HIHELP
   (D) HIQUIET

4. Discuss common legal concepts and responsibilities in health care

Matching

Use each letter only once.

1. ____ Criminal law
2. ____ Civil law
3. ____ Compliance
4. ____ Abandonment
5. ____ Standard of care
6. ____ Competence
7. ____ Liable
8. ____ Malpractice
9. ____ Good Samaritan Law
10. ____ Negligence
11. ____ Abuse
12. ____ Deposition
13. ____ Plaintiff
14. ____ Defendant
15. ____ *Res ipsa loquitur*
16. ____ *Respondeat superior*
17. ____ Subpoena

(A) Actions, or failure to act or provide proper care, resulting in unintended injury to a person

(B) Latin phrase meaning *the thing speaks for itself.* Used when a patient's injury is presented as evidence of medical negligence or wrongdoing

(C) A person accused of wrongdoing, against whom a lawsuit is filed or charges made

(D) Legally responsible

(E) A legal document that commands a person to appear in court to testify or to provide records or documents

(F) In health care, a patient's record of following the healthcare treatment plan and keeping appointments

(G) Branch of law dealing with disputes between individuals

(H) The ability to perform a task correctly

(I) A person who makes a charge of wrongdoing in court

(J) Latin term meaning *let the master answer.* Used to hold an employer liable for the actions of their employee

(K) A statement given under oath to be used as evidence in a lawsuit

(L) In health care, failure of a practitioner to provide needed care to a patient with whom a patient-practitioner relationship has been established

(M) Branch of law dealing with offenses considered to harm all of society

(N) Purposeful mistreatment that causes physical, mental, or emotional pain or injury to someone

(O) The professional standard that must be met to deliver safe and effective patient care

(P) In medicine, failure on the part of a provider to meet a professional standard of care; literal meaning is *bad practice*

(Q) A law passed to protect individuals from liability when they provide medical aid, usually in an emergency situation

Short Answer

18. What are mandated reporters?

19. Describe at least one significant difference between arbitration and mediation.

5. Discuss *consent* as it applies to health care

Matching

Use each letter only once.

1. ____ General consent
2. ____ Informed consent
3. ____ Assault
4. ____ Battery
5. ____ Emancipated minor
6. ____ Mature minor
7. ____ Implied consent

(A) Active, conscious acknowledgment that a person understands treatment they will receive and agrees to receive it

(B) A person under the age of 18 who by state law is legally considered able to make routine healthcare decisions independently

(C) Signed agreement to routine care such as examinations, laboratory tests, and blood draws

(D) The assumption that a person agrees to treatment or to a procedure; allows medical treatment to be provided in emergency situations, for example

(E) A person under 18 years of age who has been legally declared independent

(F) The intentional touching of another person without permission; can be charged if care is provided to a patient who does not consent

(G) The use of words or actions to cause another person to feel fearful of being harmed; can be charged if a patient is threatened or coerced to consent to care

6. Understand mandatory reporting requirements

Multiple Choice

1. Which of the following is an example of compliance reporting?
   (A) Reporting to the practitioner whether or not a patient has been taking her medications
   (B) Reporting to the appropriate authorities when a patient has what appears to be a gunshot wound
   (C) Reporting to the laboratory manager the number of blood draws performed in a day
   (D) Reporting to the office manager the number of insurance claims submitted in a day

Name: ______________________

2. Which of the following is a condition that must be reported?
   (A) Shingles, a viral infection common in people who have had chicken pox
   (B) Sinus infection, a frequent complication of a cold
   (C) Genital herpes, a sexually transmitted infection
   (D) A broken arm that occurred during a high school football game

3. Which of the following situations should be reported due to the medical assistant's role as a mandated reporter?
   (A) A pediatric patient has bruises and burns on his body; the accompanying parent does not allow the child to speak for himself to describe how they happened.
   (B) A 17-year-old patient in a state that allows mature minors to request vaccinations asks to receive a flu shot.
   (C) A parent tells the medical assistant in a pediatric office that their family does not allow sweets and requests that her child be offered a sticker rather than a lollipop after a visit.
   (D) An adult who is developmentally disabled is always accompanied to visits by her grandmother, who allows her granddaughter to answer questions and make choices about her care.

4. If a medical assistant suspects a patient is being abused, she should
   (A) Contact the suspected abuser and inform them that they are suspected of abuse
   (B) Watch the patient over several visits to make sure her suspicions are correct
   (C) Report it to the appropriate person immediately, following office policy/chain of command
   (D) Ask other medical assistants in the office if they have noticed anything similar

Matching

Use each letter only once.

5. ____ Suspicious injuries
6. ____ Signs associated with abuse
7. ____ Signs associated with neglect
8. ____ Signs that could indicate exploitation
9. ____ Law enforcement
10. ____ Centers for Disease Control and Prevention (CDC)
11. ____ Conflict of interest
12. ____ Examples of conditions that must be reported at regular cycles (but not immediately)
13. ____ Wounds of violence

(A) Belt buckle or strap marks; teeth marks; burns of unusual shape or in unusual locations

(B) Insulting remarks from caregiver to patient; caregiver shows hostility toward the patient and/or healthcare providers; patient's condition indicates the possibility of nonconsensual sexual activity

(C) Situation in which a person's personal interest conflicts with professional responsibilities

(D) Must be notified if danger/threat to life is suspected

(E) Gonorrhea, syphilis, and HIV

(F) Unclean body; poorly fitting clothing; unmet needs; weight loss; dehydration

(G) Gunshot wounds, knife wounds, apparent poisonings

(H) Threatening to hurt others; agitation or anxiety; signs of stress; low self-esteem; mood changes; family member/caregiver present during all conversations

(I) Must be notified of cases of anthrax, botulism, and smallpox

7. Describe incident reporting

True or False

1. _____ A medical assistant can choose whether or not to report an incident.
2. _____ Collecting a specimen from the wrong patient would be considered an incident.
3. _____ An incident report includes a description of the incident itself but does not document the response to the incident.
4. _____ Incident reports can improve the quality of healthcare services and patient safety at a facility.
5. _____ The information in an incident report should not be included in a patient's medical record.

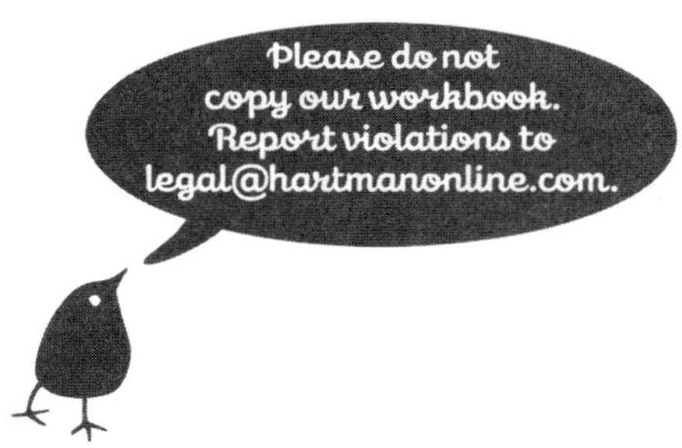

Name: ______________________________

3

Communication and Diversity

1. Define *communication*

Short Answer

1. List the three basic steps of communication.

____

____

____

____

____

2. Why is feedback an important part of communication?

____

____

____

____

____

____

3. With whom must medical assistants be able to communicate?

____

____

____

____

____

____

____

____

Multiple Choice

4. Which three things are needed for communication to take place?
   (A) Signs, symbols, and drawings
   (B) Sender, receiver, and feedback
   (C) Provider, patients, and family members
   (D) Loud voice, ability to speak, and patient's chart

5. The three-step process of communication occurs
   (A) Only once
   (B) Over and over
   (C) Only in formal meetings with the provider
   (D) In a different order every time

2. Explain verbal and nonverbal communication

Multiple Choice

1. Which of the following is an example of nonverbal communication?
   (A) Asking for a glass of water
   (B) Pointing to a glass of water
   (C) Screaming for a glass of water
   (D) Saying "I do not like water."

2. Verbal communication includes
   (A) Facial expressions
   (B) Nodding one's head
   (C) Speaking
   (D) Shrugging one's shoulders

3. Types of nonverbal communication include
   (A) Speaking
   (B) Facial expressions
   (C) Yelling
   (D) Oral reports

4. Which of the following is an example of a confusing or conflicting message (saying one thing and meaning another)?
   (A) Mr. Carter smiles happily and tells the medical assistant his new medication is helping him a lot.
   (B) Mrs. Sanchez looks like she is in pain. When the medical assistant asks her about it, Mrs. Sanchez tells her that her back has been bothering her.
   (C) Ms. Jones agrees with the medical assistant when she says it is a nice day, but Ms. Jones looks upset.
   (D) Mr. Lee will not look up from the floor. He says he is a little depressed.

5. In the previous question, how could the medical assistant clarify the confusing or conflicting message?
   (A) Tell the person that the MA knows they are not telling the truth
   (B) Ignore the conflicting message and accept what the person has said
   (C) Ask the person to repeat what they just said
   (D) State what the MA has observed and ask if the observation is correct

Short Answer

State whether each behavior below sends a positive message or a negative message to the receiver. Write P *for positive and* N *for negative.*

6. _____ Using an impatient tone
7. _____ Smiling
8. _____ Leaning forward in a chair
9. _____ Glancing repeatedly at a watch
10. _____ Sitting up straight
11. _____ Slouching
12. _____ Crossing arms in front of the body
13. _____ Listening carefully
14. _____ Nodding the head
15. _____ Rolling eyes

3. Identify barriers to communication

Crossword

Across

3. Type of terminology that may not be understood by patients or their families
5. Types of questions that should be asked because they elicit more than a "yes" or "no" answer
7. Phrases used over and over again that do not really mean anything

Down

1. Type of language, along with gestures and facial expressions, that is part of nonverbal communication
2. Being this way and taking time to listen when patients are difficult to understand helps promote better communication.
4. MAs cannot offer opinions or give this because it is not within their scope of practice.
6. MAs should not ask this when patients make statements because it often makes people feel defensive.
8. Along with profanity, these types of words and expressions should not be used by MAs.

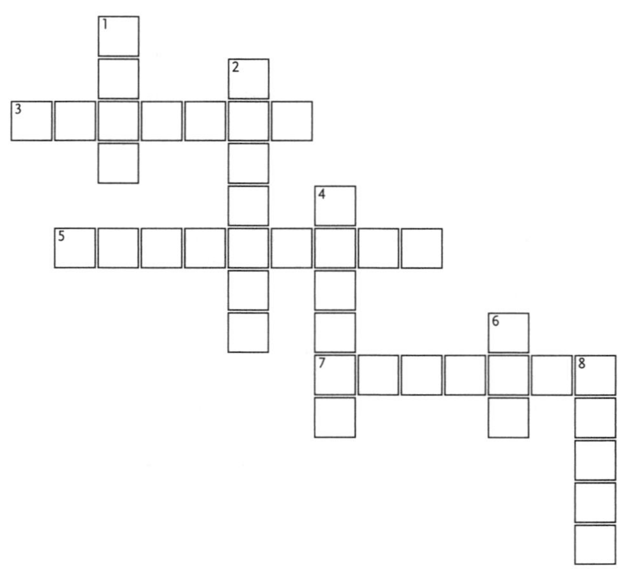

4. Define *diversity* and understand the importance of responding to diversity without bias

Matching

Use each letter only once.

1. ____ Bias
2. ____ Diversity
3. ____ Culture

(A) The variety found among people

(B) A system of learned beliefs and behaviors that are practiced by a group of people

(C) Prejudice

Short Answer

4. What are eight types of diversity medical assistants may encounter among patients?

____

____

____

____

____

5. List three things that medical assistants can do to reduce bias when working with patients.

____

____

____

____

____

6. Give an example of how one person may be influenced by many different cultures.

____

____

____

____

____

5. List guidelines for communicating with patients

Multiple Choice

Hearing Impairment

1. To best communicate with a patient who has a hearing impairment, the medical assistant should
   (A) Use short sentences and simple words
   (B) Shout
   (C) Approach the patient from behind
   (D) Raise the pitch of her voice

2. If a patient is difficult to understand, the MA should
   (A) Pretend to understand the patient so as not to hurt his feelings
   (B) Mouth the words in an exaggerated way so that the patient will mimic that behavior next time
   (C) Ask the patient to repeat what he said, and then tell the patient what the MA thinks she heard
   (D) Ask the patient to speak up

3. Which of the following settings would be best for communicating with a patient with hearing impairment?
   (A) A busy waiting room
   (B) A quiet exam room
   (C) The vital signs area, where other team members are often coming and going
   (D) The employee break room

Vision Impairment

4. Which of the following is true of patients with vision impairment?
   (A) They will all be elderly.
   (B) They will be unable to see anything at all.
   (C) They may wear contact lenses or eyeglasses.
   (D) They do not need to be told what is happening around them.

5. Where should an MA stand while talking to a patient with a vision impairment?
   (A) To the patient's side
   (B) Behind the patient
   (C) In front of the patient, facing him
   (D) In front of the patient, looking down at the patient's chart

6. When entering an examination room to care for a patient who has a visual impairment, the medical assistant should
   (A) Touch the patient, then identify herself
   (B) Be quiet so as not to startle the patient
   (C) Wait until she is very close to the patient, then touch the patient on the arm
   (D) Knock on the door and then identify herself

7. Which of the following would be appropriate for an MA to say when drawing blood from a patient with vision impairment?
   (A) "You're going to feel me touching your arm now to find a vein."
   (B) "Stay still and I'll let you know when this is over."
   (C) "I guess I don't have to tell you to look away if you don't like needles!"
   (D) "As you can see, we don't have many tubes to fill. This will be quick."

Short Answer

Mental Health Disorders

8. What should an MA avoid when communicating with a patient with a mental health disorder?

____

____

____

9. What kinds of statements should an MA use when talking to a patient with a mental health disorder?

____

____

____

10. How far away should an MA sit or stand when communicating with a patient with a mental health disorder?

____

____

Fill in the Blank

Cognitive Impairment

11. Always approach from the front, and do not ____________________.

12. Always ____________________ and use the patient's name. Continue to ____________________ as you provide care.

13. Speak slowly, using a lower ____________________ than normal. This is ____________________ and easier to understand.

14. Repeat yourself, using the same ____________________, as often as necessary.

15. Use signs, pictures, gestures, or ____________________ to help communicate as needed.

16. Ask any family member or caregiver accompanying the patient for ____________________ about communication with the patient, as appropriate.

True or False

Children

17. ____ It is important to be reassuring and to take time to help young patients manage their anxiety.

18. ____ Young children should not be allowed to sit in a parent or caregiver's lap during a medical exam.

19. ____ It is not necessary for a medical assistant to introduce himself to a pediatric patient.

20. ____ It can help for the medical assistant to lower herself physically to the child's eye level.

21. ____ An MA should always speak to the parent or caregiver rather than directly to the child.

22. ____ It is helpful to tell the child there will be a prize if they are brave and do not cry.

23. ____ When administering an injection, one helpful technique is to tell the child you will not be giving a shot, and then administer the shot when the child is not looking.

24. ____ It is never acceptable to shame or threaten a child.

Multiple Choice

Geriatric Patients

25. Which of the following is true of geriatric patients?
    (A) They all have some kind of impairment.
    (B) They are not likely to remember what happens during an exam.
    (C) They will all have similar conditions and attitudes.
    (D) They are all individuals and it is important not to make assumptions about them.

26. If a patient comes to an appointment with an adult child or other caregiver, how should the MA behave with that person?
    (A) The MA should address all communication to the child/caregiver.
    (B) The MA should not address the child/caregiver at all.
    (C) The MA should answer the child's/caregiver's questions but communicate directly with the patient.
    (D) The MA should request that the child/caregiver remain in the waiting room.

27. Which of the following is an appropriate way to address Mr. Trujillo, an elderly patient?
    (A) Gramps
    (B) Honey
    (C) Sweetie
    (D) Mr. Trujillo

Short Answer

Patients with Developmental Disabilities

State whether each behavior below is an appropriate way to communicate with patients with developmental disabilities. Write A *for appropriate and* N *for not appropriate.*

28. ____ Not describing procedures so as not to cause the patient concern

29. ____ Remaining calm and patient

30. ____ Treating adult patients with intellectual disabilities as if they were children

31. ____ Assuming the patient will not have any questions

32. ____ Asking a patient with autism spectrum disorder to please look at you while she speaks

33. ____ Watching for nonverbal cues that the patient is anxious or confused

True or False

Patients Who Speak Limited or No English

34. ____ Patients have a right to receive information about their medical care in a language they understand.

35. ____ Patients who do not understand what an MA is saying will always say that they do not understand.

36. ____ Family members or friends of the patient can be relied on for medical translation.

37. ____ It is not helpful for an MA to learn a few words or phrases of languages commonly spoken in the community where they work.

38. ____ Medical offices and facilities should have interpretation services available.

Short Answer

Patients Who Are Combative, Angry, or Inappropriate

39. List four possible causes of combative or inappropriate behavior in a patient.

____

____

____

____

40. How should a medical assistant respond if a patient makes an inappropriate or sexual comment?

____

____

____

____

____

41. What should an MA do if a patient attempts to physically strike them?

____

____

____

____

6. List ways to make communication accurate and explain how to develop effective interpersonal relationships

Multiple Choice

1. One way for an MA to be a good listener is to
   (A) Finish a patient's sentences for him to show that the MA understands what the patient is saying
   (B) Pretend that the MA understands what a patient is saying even if she does not
   (C) Restate the message in the MA's own words
   (D) Fill in any pauses to avoid awkwardness

2. Active listening involves
   (A) Focusing on the sender and giving feedback
   (B) Avoiding speaking to the patient if the MA cannot understand him
   (C) Deciding what the patient is going to say before he says it
   (D) Talking about the MA's personal problems if the patient is a good listener

3. Mrs. Velasco is a new patient who recently moved to the United States. Simon, a medical assistant, is taking her medical, family, and social history. She tells Simon that she is having a difficult time adjusting to life in the US and does not feel like she understands American customs. What would be the best response by Simon?
   (A) Give her advice about how to fit in better with American culture
   (B) Tell her this really isn't what he was asking about and request that she stick with the subject of her medical history
   (C) Tell her that he can imagine how difficult the move must have been for her and ask her if she has a support system to help her with these challenges
   (D) Speed up the questions so he can reduce his feelings of discomfort

4. When patients report symptoms or feelings, the best response by the MA is to
   (A) Interrupt to ask for more details
   (B) Give medical advice
   (C) Avoid speaking or responding
   (D) Listen and then ask for more information

5. Which of the following statements reflects a way for a medical assistant to have positive relationships with patients?
   (A) The MA should fold her arms in front of her while patients are talking.
   (B) The MA should tell patients she knows exactly how they feel, so patients will feel like they have something in common.
   (C) The MA should ignore a patient's request if she knows she cannot fulfill it.
   (D) The MA should be empathetic and try to understand what patients are going through.

6. Mr. Vernon is an elderly patient who has terminal cancer. He is telling Katie, a medical assistant, that he is very depressed about dying. He feels he has left many things unfinished. Hearing this makes Katie uncomfortable. Which of the following would be the best response by Katie?
   (A) She should try to ignore what he is saying until he changes the subject.
   (B) She should try to interest him in a brighter subject.
   (C) She should listen to him and ask questions when appropriate.
   (D) She should try to relate to him by telling him she knows just how he feels.

7. Rick, a medical assistant, is going through a difficult time personally and has been late for work every day for more than a week. He arrives before the provider arrives, but has not been on time to help with opening the office, which is part of his job. He has been texting Jake and asking him to clock in for him and cover his morning duties. Which of the following responses from Jake demonstrates an assertive communication style?
   (A) "I've covered for you enough already. Just get it together and come in when you're supposed to."
   (B) "I know you've been having a rough time and I'm sorry. I've realized covering for you isn't honest, though, and it means I can't do my work. I can't do this anymore."
   (C) "I'll do it today but if you ask me one more time I'm telling the doctor."
   (D) "Sure. I guess I can open for you again a few more times."

7. Explain objective and subjective information and describe how to observe and report accurately

Short Answer

For each of the following, decide whether it is an objective observation (you can see, hear, smell, or touch it) or a subjective observation (the patient must tell you about it). Write O for objective and S for subjective.

1. _____ Skin rash
2. _____ Crying
3. _____ Rapid pulse
4. _____ Headache
5. _____ Nausea
6. _____ Vomiting
7. _____ Swelling
8. _____ Cloudy urine
9. _____ Wheezing
10. _____ Feeling sad
11. _____ Red area on skin
12. _____ Fever
13. _____ Dizziness
14. _____ Chest pain
15. _____ Toothache
16. _____ Coughing
17. _____ Fruity breath
18. _____ Itchy arm

Labeling

Looking at the diagram, list examples of observations using each sense.

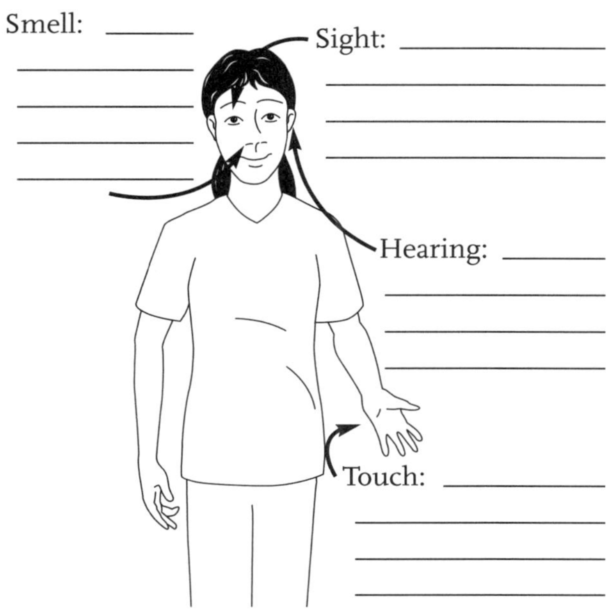

Name: ______________________________

8. Explain how to communicate with other healthcare workers

Multiple Choice

1. When giving information about a patient to other members of the care team, a medical assistant should
   (A) Use a code name to discuss the patient if other patients are present
   (B) Make a possible diagnosis of the patient's condition
   (C) Share information with anyone who asks about the patient's condition
   (D) Make sure that she respects the patient's right to privacy

2. One health professional who is able to give a patient's family and friends information about any new diagnoses is a(n)
   (A) Physician
   (B) Medical assistant
   (C) Coding and billing specialist
   (D) Lab technician

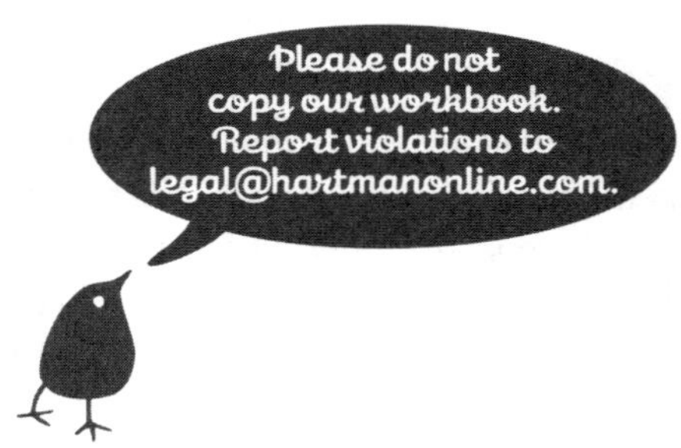

4

Psychology and Human Needs and Development

1. Identify basic human needs and describe holistic care

Short Answer

1. List five basic physiological needs that all humans have.

____

____

____

____

____

____

2. List six psychosocial needs that humans have.

____

____

____

____

____

____

3. Complete your own hierarchy of needs below. Some of the examples have already been completed for you.

Maslow's Hierarchy of Needs

Needs

(A) Need for self-actualization

(B) Need for self-esteem

(C) Need for love

(D) Safety and security needs

(E) Physiological needs

Examples of Needs

(A) I need the chance to learn new things.

(B) I need to know that I am doing a good job.

(C) ______________________________

____

(D) ______________________________

____

(E) ______________________________

____

Short Answer

4. In your own words, briefly define holistic care.

____

____

____

____

2. Describe the stages of human growth and development and identify common disorders for each stage

True or False

1. ____ A child takes three years from birth to be able to move around, communicate basic needs, and feed himself.

2. ____ Infant physical development moves from the hands to the head.

3. ____ Caregivers should encourage infants to stand as soon as they can hold their heads up.

Name: ________________________________

4. _____ Putting an infant to sleep on its back can reduce the risk of sudden infant death syndrome (SIDS).

5. _____ Tantrums are common among toddlers.

6. _____ The best way to deal with tantrums is to give the toddler what he wants.

7. _____ Preschool children are too young to know right from wrong.

8. _____ Children learn to speak between the ages of 3 and 5.

9. _____ From the ages of 5 to 10, children learn to get along with each other.

10. _____ School-age children (5 to 10 years) develop cognitively and socially.

11. _____ Preadolescents are often easy to get along with and are able to handle more responsibility than they were before.

12. _____ Puberty is the stage of growth when secondary sex characteristics, such as body hair, appear.

13. _____ Most adolescents do not feel that peer acceptance is important.

14. _____ Adolescents may be moody due to changing hormones and body image concerns.

15. _____ Eating disorders are difficult to deal with but cannot be life-threatening.

16. _____ Due to changes they are experiencing, adolescents may become depressed and may attempt suicide.

17. _____ By 18 years of age, most young adults have stopped developing physically, psychologically, and socially.

18. _____ One developmental task that most young adults undertake is to choose an occupation or career.

19. _____ A "midlife crisis" is a period of unrest when a person has an unconscious desire for change and fulfillment of unmet goals.

20. _____ Middle-aged adults usually do not experience any physical changes due to aging.

21. _____ Menopause is a condition that occurs in young women when the ovaries begin to secrete hormones.

22. _____ By the time a person reaches late adulthood, he must adjust to the effects of aging.

3. Explain developmental disabilities

Crossword

Across

2. Intensely focused interests, difficulty imagining other people's thought processes or emotions, and a preference not to make this kind of contact are differences resulting from autism spectrum disorder.
4. Split spine
5. Muscle coordination and nerves are affected by this disorder.

Down

1. Most common developmental disorder
3. Developmental disability that causes a small skull, flattened nose, and shorter fingers

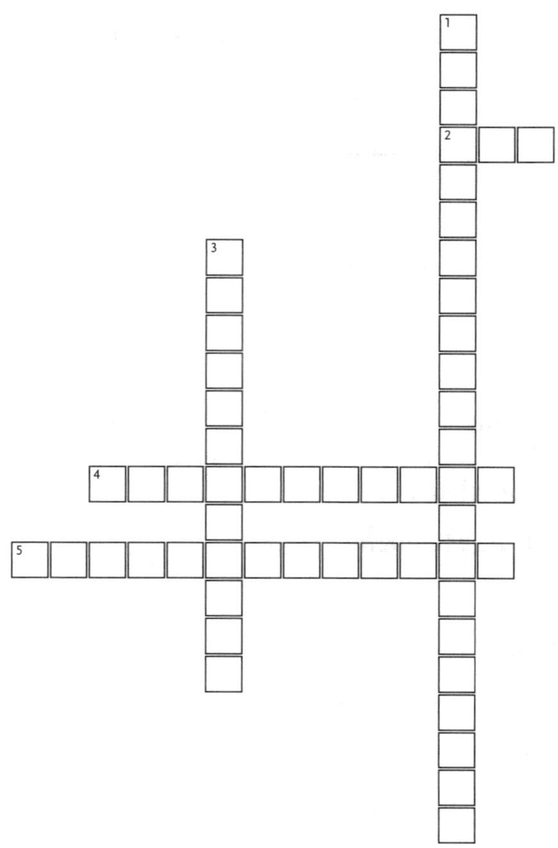

4. Identify seven characteristics of mental health and explain the connection between mental and physical wellness

Short Answer

1. Define *mental health.*

2. List seven characteristics of a person who is mentally healthy.

5. Define *stress* and *stressors* and discuss the psychological effects of stress

Short Answer

1. What are some situations that make you experience stress? How do you react when you are stressed?

6. Identify and define common defense mechanisms

Short Answer

Read each description below and identify the defense mechanism that is being used.

1. When Aaron's mother yells at him for breaking a vase in the living room, he goes into his room and yells at his stuffed bear.

2. When Gia was 10, she was very badly injured in a car accident. She was in the hospital for almost three months, but now she tries not to think about that time.

3. When Marco accuses his little sister Ana of having a crush on the boy who sits next to her in class, she blushes and cries, "I do not!"

____

____

____

____

4. When Esther was 42, her husband died of lung cancer. After his death, she got out the quilt she used to sleep with as a child and curled up in bed with it for days.

____

____

____

____

5. Wayne is fixing a leaky sink in the bathroom. When his wife teases him about taking a long time to fix it, he replies, "It's not my fault. I can't concentrate on anything with you bothering me all the time."

____

____

____

____

6. Martin's girlfriend promised to go out with him on Thursday night, but she forgot and made plans with her sister instead. Martin is annoyed, but does not say anything to her. When he goes out with his friends that night, he tells them that she is mad at him.

____

____

____

____

7. List the signs of substance abuse and discuss other addiction disorders

Multiple Choice

1. Circle any of the following substances that can be abused:
   (A) Alcohol
   (B) Cigarettes
   (C) Decongestants
   (D) Diet aids
   (E) Illegal drugs
   (F) Glue
   (G) Paint
   (H) Prescription medicine

2. A patient's behavior seems unusual to Stephanie, a medical assistant. During intake for a 9:00 a.m. appointment the patient gets upset several times, and her eyes are red. Stephanie thinks she can smell alcohol on the patient's breath. What would be the best response from Stephanie?
   (A) Confront the patient about what she has noticed
   (B) Contact Alcoholics Anonymous to get advice on how to handle the situation
   (C) Document her observations and report them to the provider
   (D) While taking the patient's history, ask how long she's had an alcohol problem

3. Which of the following statements about chemical dependency is true?
   (A) Chemical dependency always involves use of an illegal substance.
   (B) Recovery from chemical dependency is as simple as stopping use of the substance.
   (C) Chemical dependency may cause a person to require more of the substance to get the same effect.
   (D) Chemical dependency primarily affects a person emotionally.

8. Describe causes and types of mental health disorders

True or False

1. ____ Mental health disorders are not at all similar to physical health disorders.
2. ____ Intense stress may cause a mental health disorder to arise or worsen.
3. ____ Signs of mental health disorders are unlike anything mentally healthy people ever experience.
4. ____ Mental health disorders can be caused by substance abuse or a chemical imbalance.
5. ____ The building blocks of mental health are self-respect and self-worth.
6. ____ Traumatic experiences early in life do not cause mental health disorders.
7. ____ Mental health disorders cannot be inherited.
8. ____ Mental health disorders are not known to cause inappropriate behavior.
9. ____ Physical factors related to the brain may make a mental health disorder more likely to develop.

Multiple Choice

10. Uneasiness, worry, or fear, often about a situation or condition, is called
    (A) Anxiety
    (B) Withdrawal
    (C) Fatigue
    (D) Apathy
11. An intense, irrational fear of or anxiety about an object, place, or situation is called a
    (A) Depressive episode
    (B) Delusion
    (C) Phobia
    (D) Hallucination
12. Postpartum ________ may occur after a woman gives birth.
    (A) Anxiety
    (B) Apathy
    (C) Irritability
    (D) Depression
13. Which of the following disorders is characterized by recurring intrusive behavior or thoughts?
    (A) Generalized anxiety disorder
    (B) Posttraumatic stress disorder
    (C) Obsessive-compulsive disorder
    (D) Schizophrenia
14. A persistent false belief, such as a person believing that someone else is controlling his thoughts, is a
    (A) Defense mechanism
    (B) Delusion
    (C) Phobia
    (D) Hallucination

9. Discuss the psychological effects of chronic and serious illness

Multiple Choice

1. Which of the following is a common response to the diagnosis of a chronic or serious illness?
   (A) A *Why me?* reaction
   (B) Lack of concern or interest
   (C) Violence against the MA or provider
   (D) Relief and contentment
2. Which of the following may reduce the stress caused by chronic illness?
   (A) Constant research into the illness
   (B) Maintaining connections with family and friends
   (C) Refusing help, which proves independence
   (D) Working and engaging in other activities so intensely that there is no time to think about the illness

Name: ______________________________

3. What reaction is common among parents when a child is diagnosed with a serious illness?
   (A) Anger at the child
   (B) Lack of concern or interest
   (C) Guilt or worry that they caused the condition
   (D) A decision to cut ties with the medical provider who made the diagnosis

10. Understand end-of-life concerns and the stages of grief

True or False

1. _____ A terminal illness will eventually cause death.

2. _____ Older people or those with terminal illnesses rarely have time to prepare for death.

3. _____ Preparing for death is a process that affects the dying person's emotions and behavior.

4. _____ All people with terminal illnesses will pass through each stage described by Dr. Kübler-Ross.

5. _____ People who are dying may move back and forth between the stages of the grief process.

Multiple Choice

Read each scenario below and choose which stage of grief the person described is experiencing.

6. Mr. Cane was told two years ago that a tumor in his brain was inoperable and would eventually be fatal. Since that time, he has visited many specialists. Despite receiving the same diagnosis from every doctor, he continues to seek further opinions, insisting that each doctor try to remove the tumor. Which stage of grief is Mr. Cane in?
   (A) Denial
   (B) Anger
   (C) Bargaining
   (D) Depression
   (E) Acceptance

7. Mrs. Williams is dying of heart disease. During an appointment at her doctor's office, Mrs. Williams lashes out at Annie, a medical assistant. She tells Annie that she is a dumb girl who is wasting her life and does not deserve the many years she has left to live. Which stage of grief is Mrs. Williams in?
   (A) Denial
   (B) Anger
   (C) Bargaining
   (D) Depression
   (E) Acceptance

8. Mr. Lopez is dying of AIDS. He has called all of his friends to say goodbye and has discussed at length with his family the kind of memorial service he would like them to arrange. What stage of grief is Mr. Lopez in?
   (A) Denial
   (B) Anger
   (C) Bargaining
   (D) Depression
   (E) Acceptance

9. Ms. Corke has always been lively and happy. Since she learned that she has Lou Gehrig's disease, however, her mood has changed drastically. Although she is still healthy enough to do activities, during intake for a doctor's appointment she reports to the medical assistant that she rarely leaves her home or even changes out of her night-clothes. Which stage of grief is Ms. Corke in?
   (A) Denial
   (B) Anger
   (C) Bargaining
   (D) Depression
   (E) Acceptance

5

Infection Prevention and Control

1. Define *infection prevention* and discuss types of infections

Matching

Use each letter only once.

1. _____ Healthcare-associated infection
2. _____ Infection
3. _____ Infection prevention
4. _____ Localized infection
5. _____ Microorganism/microbe
6. _____ Pathogen
7. _____ Systemic infection

(A) Set of methods practiced in healthcare facilities to prevent and control the spread of disease

(B) A harmful microorganism

(C) An infection acquired in a healthcare setting during the delivery of medical care

(D) A small living thing that is only visible under a microscope

(E) An infection that travels through the bloodstream and is spread throughout the body

(F) Occurs when pathogens invade and multiply within the body

(G) An infection that is limited to a specific location in the body

2. Describe the chain of infection

Multiple Choice

1. The following are necessary links in the chain of infection. Which link is broken by wearing gloves, thus preventing the spread of disease?
   (A) Reservoir (place where the pathogen lives and grows)
   (B) Mode of transmission (a way for the disease to spread)
   (C) Susceptible host (person who is likely to get the disease)
   (D) Portal of exit (body opening that allows pathogens to leave)

2. The following are necessary links in the chain of infection. By getting a vaccination for hepatitis B, which link will a person affect to prevent him from getting this disease?
   (A) Reservoir (place where the pathogen lives and grows)
   (B) Mode of transmission (a way for the disease to spread)
   (C) Susceptible host (person who is likely to get the disease)
   (D) Portal of exit (body opening that allows pathogens to leave)

3. Handwashing with regular soap and water is one form of
   (A) Medical asepsis
   (B) Personal protective equipment
   (C) Surgical asepsis
   (D) Sterile technique

4. In what type of environment do microorganisms grow best?
   (A) In a warm, moist place
   (B) In a bright place
   (C) In a cool, dry place
   (D) In a frozen place

3. Explain Standard Precautions

True or False

1. ____ Following Standard Precautions means treating blood and other body fluids, nonintact skin, and mucous membranes as if they were infected.
2. ____ Under Standard Precautions, body fluids do not include saliva.
3. ____ A medical assistant can usually tell if someone has an infectious illness just by looking at him.
4. ____ A medical assistant should wash her hands before donning (putting on) gloves.
5. ____ A medical assistant should carefully recap used syringes before putting them in a biohazard container.
6. ____ Removing sutures is one task that requires an MA to wear gloves.
7. ____ A mask and goggles may need to be worn when emptying a bedpan.
8. ____ Biomedical/biohazard waste that is not sharp should be discarded in a regular trash bag.

Multiple Choice

9. Standard Precautions should be practiced
   (A) Only on patients who look like they have a bloodborne disease
   (B) On every single patient a medical assistant encounters
   (C) Only on patients who request that the medical assistant follow them
   (D) Only on patients who have tuberculosis

10. Standard Precautions include the following measures:
   (A) Washing hands after taking off gloves but not before putting on gloves
   (B) Wearing gloves if there is a possibility of coming into contact with blood or other body fluids, mucous membranes, or broken skin
   (C) Touching body fluids with bare hands
   (D) Disposing of sharps in plastic bags

11. Which of the following is true of both Standard Precautions and Transmission-Based Precautions?
   (A) They are different names for the same thing.
   (B) They stop an infected person from giving off pathogens.
   (C) They can prevent pathogens from an infected patient from infecting others.
   (D) They vary by state and facility.

12. How should sharps be discarded?
   (A) Sharps should be placed in blue recycling containers.
   (B) Sharps should be placed in break room trash containers.
   (C) Sharps should be placed inside used gloves and then put in hazardous waste bags.
   (D) Sharps should be placed in puncture-resistant biohazard containers.

13. The Occupational Safety and Health Administration (OSHA) is a federal government agency that protects workers from
   (A) Unfair employment practices
   (B) Sexual harassment
   (C) Workplace violence
   (D) Hazards on the job

4. Explain hand hygiene and identify when to wash hands

Multiple Choice

1. A medical assistant will come into contact with microorganisms
   (A) Only in public areas of the medical facility where she works
   (B) Only during direct contact with patients
   (C) Only during care that involves touching a patient
   (D) Every time the MA touches something

2. Centers for Disease Control and Prevention (CDC) defines hand hygiene as
   (A) Handwashing with soap and water or using alcohol-based hand rubs
   (B) Using only alcohol-based hand rubs when hands are visibly soiled
   (C) Rinsing hands with cold water
   (D) Not washing hands more than once per day

3. Alcohol-based hand rubs are used
   (A) With water for maximum effectiveness
   (B) When facilities have run out of antimicrobial soap
   (C) To prevent dry, cracked skin
   (D) In addition to washing with soap and water

4. Why should a medical assistant not wear artificial nails to work?
   (A) Patients may not like them.
   (B) They may be damaged during patient care.
   (C) They harbor bacteria and increase risk of contamination.
   (D) They may be torn or damaged by frequent handwashing.

5. How long should a medical assistant use friction when lathering and washing her hands?
   (A) 2 minutes
   (B) 5 seconds
   (C) 18 seconds
   (D) 20 seconds

5. Discuss the use of personal protective equipment (PPE)

Short Answer

Place a check mark (✓) next to the tasks that require a medical assistant to wear gloves.

1. ____ Contact with body fluids
2. ____ When the MA may touch blood
3. ____ Taking a patient's blood pressure
4. ____ Answering the telephone
5. ____ Assisting with a surgical procedure
6. ____ Collecting a copayment
7. ____ Collecting a sputum specimen (a specimen of mucus coughed up by the patient)
8. ____ Drawing blood
9. ____ Putting ointment in a patient's eye

Multiple Choice

10. What type of PPE may be needed when caring for a patient with a respiratory illness?
    (A) Eyeglasses and mask
    (B) Mask and foot covering
    (C) Eyeglasses and gloves
    (D) Mask and goggles

11. What type of PPE is used most often by healthcare workers?
    (A) Gloves
    (B) Mask
    (C) Face shield
    (D) Goggles

12. How many times can a gown be worn before it needs to be discarded?
    (A) One time
    (B) Two times
    (C) Three times
    (D) Four times

Name: ______________________________

13. If blood or body fluids may be splashed or sprayed into the eye area, proper protection for the eyes is
    (A) Eyeglasses
    (B) Mask
    (C) Sunglasses
    (D) Goggles

Short Answer

After Zoe washes her hands, she will put on her PPE. She is going into an area in which she needs to use Transmission-Based Precautions, so she will wear a gown, a mask, and goggles in addition to her gloves. Read the steps she takes and write down anything she does incorrectly.

14. First Zoe puts on her gown. She holds it out in front of her and shakes it open. She slips her arms into the sleeves and then ties the neck ties in a secure knot so that it will not come untied while she is working. She reaches behind her and, making sure all of her clothing is covered, secures the gown at the waist.

____

____

____

____

____

____

____

____

15. Zoe then puts on her mask. Being careful not to touch the mask where it touches her face, she ties the bottom strings first and then the top strings. She then puts on her goggles, making sure they fit snugly over her eyeglasses.

____

____

____

____

____

____

____

____

16. Zoe is right-handed, so she puts on her right glove first. She then uses her gloved hand to put on her other glove. She holds her hands out in front of her to smooth out the folds in the gloves. She looks closely at the gloves for tears or holes. She sees an area that is discolored, but it is very small, so she decides to wear the glove anyway. She pulls the sleeves of her gown over the cuffs of the gloves and is ready to get to work.

____

____

____

____

____

____

____

____

____

Short Answer

17. What is the correct order for donning (putting on) PPE (gloves, mask, gown, goggles)?

1st ______________________________

2nd ______________________________

3rd ______________________________

4th ______________________________

18. What is the correct order for doffing (removing) PPE (gloves, mask, gown, goggles)?

1st ______________________________

2nd ______________________________

3rd ______________________________

4th ______________________________

19. Which type of PPE must be removed AFTER exiting the patient's room?

____

____

6. Explain Transmission-Based Precautions

Short Answer

List the type of precaution being described in each phrase below. Use an A for Airborne Precautions, a C for Contact Precautions, and a D for Droplet Precautions. Each letter may be used more than once.

1. ____ Transmission can occur when touching a contaminated area on the patient's body.
2. ____ Used when there is a risk of spreading an infection by direct contact with a person or object
3. ____ Used to guard against tuberculosis
4. ____ Covering the nose and mouth with a tissue when a person sneezes or coughs and washing hands immediately after sneezing are parts of these precautions.
5. ____ Helps prevent the spread of *Clostridioides difficile* (*C. diff*) and conjunctivitis
6. ____ Used when the microorganisms are spread by droplets in the air that travel only short distances (normally not more than 6 feet)
7. ____ Microorganisms can be spread by coughing, sneezing, talking, laughing, or suctioning.
8. ____ Helps prevent the spread of illnesses transmitted through the air
9. ____ Helps protect against transmission of influenza
10. ____ May require the use of a special mask, such as an N95 or HEPA mask

Multiple Choice

11. Transmission-Based Precautions are used
    (A) With every patient a medical assistant encounters
    (B) In addition to Standard Precautions
    (C) Instead of Standard Precautions
    (D) When an MA decides that they are appropriate for particular patients

12. Which of the following is true of equipment that is not disposable and is used in caring for multiple patients?
    (A) It can never be used on patients with known infectious illnesses.
    (B) It can only be used by physicians and other licensed medical professionals.
    (C) It must be disinfected on a daily basis.
    (D) It must be disinfected after each use.

13. Which of the following is true of wearing PPE while caring for patients in isolation?
    (A) Medical assistants will have to decide for themselves which PPE they must wear while caring for patients in isolation.
    (B) Medical assistants should remove most PPE before exiting an isolation room.
    (C) Medical assistants will always wear the same PPE while caring for all patients in isolation.
    (D) Medical assistants should remove all PPE after exiting an isolation room.

14. When a patient is in isolation,
    (A) She should be avoided
    (B) Medical assistants will be unable to perform care for her
    (C) She needs to feel that her feelings are understood by care team members
    (D) Medical assistants should not practice Standard Precautions

Name: ____________________

7. Define *bloodborne pathogens* and describe two major bloodborne diseases

Multiple Choice

1. Bloodborne diseases can be transmitted by
   (A) Infected blood entering the bloodstream
   (B) Hugging a person with a bloodborne disease
   (C) Being in the same room as a person with a bloodborne disease
   (D) Exercising with a person who has a bloodborne disease

2. In a healthcare setting, the most common way to be infected by a bloodborne disease is by
   (A) Contact with infected blood or certain body fluids
   (B) Sharing contaminated needles between patients
   (C) Being in the same room as a patient with a bloodborne disease
   (D) Sexual contact with an infected patient

3. How does the human immunodeficiency virus (HIV) affect the body?
   (A) It cuts off blood supply to the brain.
   (B) It causes inadequate nutritional intake by damaging the gastrointestinal system.
   (C) It causes diabetes in otherwise healthy people.
   (D) It weakens the immune system so that the body cannot fight infection.

4. Which of the following is true of hepatitis B (HBV)?
   (A) HBV is caused by fecal-oral contamination.
   (B) There is no vaccine for HBV.
   (C) HBV is caused by jaundice.
   (D) HBV can be transmitted through blood or needles that are contaminated with the virus.

5. Employers must offer a free vaccine to protect medical assistants from
   (A) AIDS
   (B) Hepatitis B
   (C) Hepatitis C
   (D) All bloodborne diseases

8. Explain OSHA's Bloodborne Pathogens Standard and the Needlestick Safety and Prevention Act

Multiple Choice

1. The Bloodborne Pathogens Standard is a law that requires that
   (A) Healthcare employers must have a written exposure control plan designed to eliminate or reduce employee exposure to infectious material
   (B) Healthcare employers must only accept patients who are free of bloodborne diseases
   (C) Healthcare employers must charge employees a discounted fee for hepatitis B vaccinations
   (D) Healthcare employers must disclose information about patients' bloodborne diseases to the public

2. Which of the following does OSHA consider a significant exposure?
   (A) MA is stuck by a needle
   (B) Patient makes a complaint against an MA
   (C) MA does not discard their PPE properly
   (D) MA was recently diagnosed with cancer

3. Which of the following is an example of the type of engineering control required by the Needlestick Safety and Prevention Act?
   (A) An N95 respirator
   (B) An eyewash station
   (C) A hinged or sliding needle sheath
   (D) A sharps container

4. According to OSHA, employers must give all employees, patients, and visitors ________ to use when needed.
   (A) Syringe caps
   (B) Safety Data Sheets (SDS)
   (C) PPE
   (D) Medical charts

5. Why is it important for an employee to report any potential exposures immediately?
   (A) So that the employee can be terminated to avoid infecting others
   (B) To avoid any appearance of negligence on the part of the facility
   (C) To protect the employee's health and the health of others
   (D) So that the employee can warn patients of a possible epidemic

9. List guidelines for handling equipment and specimens

Matching

Use each letter only once.

1. _____ Clean
2. _____ Dirty
3. _____ Disinfection
4. _____ Sterilization

(A) A cleaning measure that destroys all microorganisms, including those that form spores

(B) A process that destroys most, but not all, pathogens

(C) In health care, objects that have not been contaminated with pathogens

(D) In health care, objects that have been contaminated with pathogens

Multiple Choice

5. Where should specimen tubes and containers be placed for transport?
   (A) In the MA's pocket
   (B) In a puncture-proof sharps receptacle
   (C) In a plastic zipper bag
   (D) In a biohazard bag

6. After collecting a specimen from a patient, what must the MA always do before calling the next patient to the examination room?
   (A) Ask the provider's permission
   (B) Clean and disinfect all surfaces
   (C) Run required tests on the specimen
   (D) Ask the patient to clean everything they touched

7. Where should needles or sharps used in specimen collection be placed?
   (A) In with the specimen
   (B) In a separate biohazard bag
   (C) In the trash
   (D) In a puncture-proof sharps receptacle

10. List employer and employee responsibilities for infection prevention

Short Answer

Read the following and mark ER *for employer or* EE *for employee to show who is responsible for infection prevention.*

1. _____ Immediately report any exposure to infection, blood, or body fluids.
2. _____ Provide PPE for use and train how to properly use it.
3. _____ Follow all facility policies and procedures.
4. _____ Take advantage of the free hepatitis B vaccination.
5. _____ Provide continuing in-service education about infection prevention.
6. _____ Establish infection prevention procedures and an exposure control plan.
7. _____ Follow patient care plans and assignments.
8. _____ Participate in continuing in-service education programs covering infection prevention.
9. _____ Use PPE as indicated or as appropriate.
10. _____ Provide free hepatitis B vaccinations.

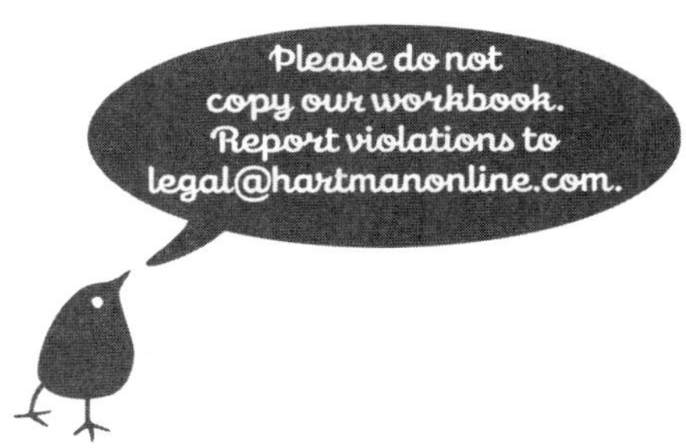

Name: ______________________________

Name: ______________________________

6

Safety, Emergency Care, and Disaster Preparation

1. Demonstrate how to recognize and respond to medical emergencies

Crossword

Across

4. Being mentally alert and having awareness of surroundings, sensations, and thoughts
6. In addition to completing an incident report, action the MA should take after the emergency is over

Down

1. Type of wound that is considered a medical emergency
2. After assessing the situation, what the person who responds to a medical emergency must assess
3. In addition to checking for danger, noticing this is part of assessing the situation during a medical emergency.
5. The opposite of opinions; they need to be reported when documenting an emergency

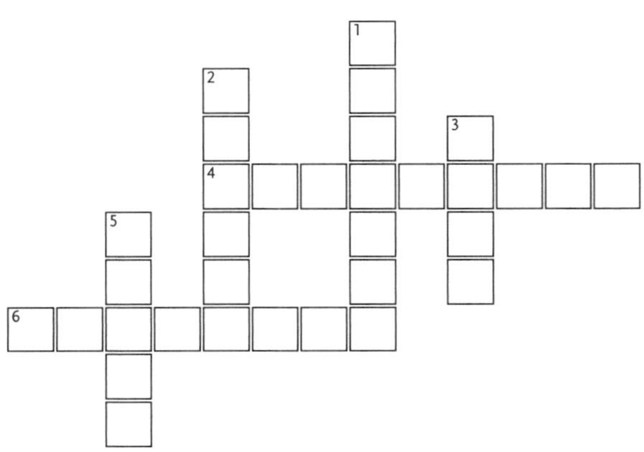

2. Demonstrate knowledge of first aid procedures

Multiple Choice

1. First aid refers to
   (A) Care given by the first people to respond to an emergency
   (B) The person with the highest level of medical training who responds to the emergency
   (C) Any person the victim has given permission to treat him during an emergency
   (D) The first person to give consent to medical professionals for treating the victim

2. If an emergency occurs, the MA should immediately notify
   (A) The patient's family
   (B) The provider
   (C) Anyone in the waiting room who arrived with the patient
   (D) The patient's religious leader

3. How can someone usually tell if a person is choking?
   (A) The choking victim will tell the person.
   (B) The choking victim will ask for food.
   (C) The choking victim will put his hands to his throat.
   (D) The choking victim will vomit.

4. Where should the hands be placed to give abdominal thrusts?
   (A) Under the person's arms and around their waist
   (B) Under the person's arms and around their chest
   (C) Over the person's shoulders and around their neck
   (D) Under the person's arms and around their pelvis

5. How does a rescuer get consent to give a choking victim abdominal thrusts?
   (A) The rescuer asks the victim's spouse to sign a consent form.
   (B) The rescuer asks the provider, "May I treat this person?"
   (C) The rescuer asks an attorney first.
   (D) The rescuer asks the victim, "Are you choking?"

6. Signs of shock include
   (A) Pale, bluish, or discolored skin
   (B) Lack of thirst
   (C) Being asleep
   (D) Relaxation

7. If a medical assistant suspects that a patient is having a heart attack, she should
   (A) Give the patient something cold to drink
   (B) Loosen the clothing around the patient's neck
   (C) Encourage the patient to walk around
   (D) Leave the patient alone to rest

8. To control bleeding, an MA should
   (A) Use her bare hands to stop it
   (B) Lower the wound below the level of the heart
   (C) Hold a thick pad or clean cloth against the wound and press down hard
   (D) Give the patient an aspirin

9. Which kind of burn involves just the outer layer of skin?
   (A) First-degree (superficial)
   (B) Second-degree (partial-thickness)
   (C) Third-degree (full-thickness)
   (D) Fourth-degree (deep-thickness)

10. To treat a minor burn, the MA should
    (A) Use antibacterial ointment
    (B) Use grease, such as butter
    (C) Use ice water
    (D) Use cool, clean water

11. If a patient faints, the MA should
    (A) Lower the patient to the floor
    (B) Position the patient on his stomach
    (C) Perform CPR
    (D) Help the patient stand up immediately

12. If a patient has a nosebleed, what should be the first step that the MA takes?
    (A) Report and document the incident.
    (B) Apply pressure consistently until the bleeding stops.
    (C) Apply a cool cloth on the back of the neck, the forehead, or the upper lip.
    (D) Tell the patient to remain in a sitting position.

13. When a patient is first experiencing signs of insulin reaction (hypoglycemia), what needs to happen?
    (A) Food that can be rapidly absorbed or a glucose tablet should be consumed.
    (B) The person should lie down and be left alone to rest.
    (C) The MA should give the patient his diabetes medication.
    (D) CPR should be started.

14. Which of the following is true of assisting a patient who is having a seizure?
    (A) The MA should give the patient water to drink.
    (B) The MA should hold the patient down if he is shaking severely.
    (C) The MA should move furniture away to prevent injury to the patient.
    (D) The MA should open the patient's mouth to move the tongue to the side.

15. Why is a quick response to a suspected stroke/CVA critical?
    (A) A quick response means that the facility will not be liable.
    (B) Early treatment may be able to reduce the severity of the stroke.
    (C) Patients will be able to say their goodbyes to family members.
    (D) Patients will experience no problems at all if there is a quick response.

16. If a patient falls, the MA should
    (A) Wait until the end of the day to report the fall
    (B) Ask the patient to get up to see if she can walk
    (C) Notify the provider
    (D) Move the patient to the bed

3. Discuss workplace safety and identify OSHA's categories of common hazards

Fill in the Blank

1. ____________________ staff members, including ____________________, are responsible for safety in a facility.
2. Bloodborne pathogens are one significant ____________________ MAs may encounter.
3. Physical hazards include poor ____________________ practices. They also include exposure to ____________________ or ____________________.
4. The ____________________ of chairs for drawing blood, the location of ____________________ and supplies, and the amount of space in a(n) ____________________ can all affect safety.
5. Healthcare workers should review and practice safety responses often so that they become ____________________.

4. Describe regulations related to safety practices and explain the Safety Data Sheet

Matching

Match each category to one of the examples below. Use each letter only once.

1. ____ Work practices
2. ____ Engineering controls
3. ____ PPE
4. ____ Administrative controls

(A) Devices, such as needle sheaths, that prevent workers from coming into contact with hazards

(B) Equipment, such as gloves, used when contact with hazards is likely

(C) Practices, such as using the least caustic cleaning agent, that change how work is done to limit exposure to hazards

(D) Policies and procedures, such as ways to handle blood or body fluids, that employers put in place to limit possible dangers

Multiple Choice

5. Which of the following is included on a Safety Data Sheet (SDS)?
   (A) Chemical ingredients and dangers
   (B) Correct response to patient abuse
   (C) Fire evacuation procedures
   (D) Safe handling information for blood specimens
6. Employers must
   (A) Keep SDS information confidential from employees
   (B) Terminate employees who do not know how to use an SDS
   (C) Have an SDS for every chemical used
   (D) Edit an SDS if they do not agree with what is listed

5. Explain the principles of body mechanics

Labeling

Complete the illustration by labeling each part with the words listed below.

Alignment

Base of support

Center of gravity

Fulcrum

Lever

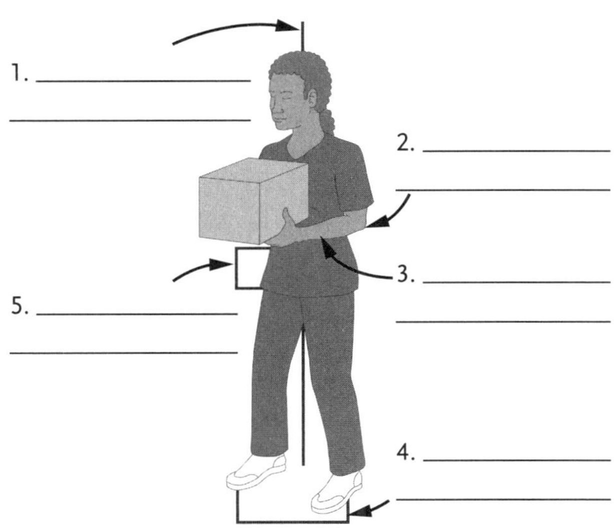

Name: ______________________________

True or False

6. ____ Healthcare workers are at risk for back injuries and strain.
7. ____ Using proper body mechanics can help save energy and prevent injury.
8. ____ When lifting an object, it is safer to hold it far away from the body.
9. ____ Feet should be pointed toward the object that a person is lifting.
10. ____ Keeping the feet close together gives the body the best base of support and keeps a person more stable.
11. ____ A high center of gravity gives a more stable base of support.
12. ____ Knees should be bent when lifting an object.

6. Describe guidelines for responding to common hazards and disasters

Short Answer

1. According to the CDC, what should be developed in a workplace to avoid danger?

____

____

2. What should an MA do if he notices a possible hazard in the workplace?

____

____

3. List two types of chemicals MAs regularly use on the job.

____

____

4. Why should dried blood or other body fluids not be scraped off of a surface or floor?

____

____

5. What are two ways for medical assistants to protect themselves against radiation exposure?

____

____

____

____

____

____

6. What should an MA do about damaged or malfunctioning equipment?

____

____

____

____

____

____

7. PASS is an acronym that stands for
   P: ____________
   A: ____________
   S: ____________
   S: ____________

8. RACE is an acronym that stands for
   R: ____________
   A: ____________
   C: ____________
   E: ____________

9. Explain the fire safety technique *stop, drop, and roll.*

____

____

____

____

____

Name: ______________________________

Multiple Choice

10. A general guideline to follow during a disaster is to
    (A) Turn off your phone to save battery
    (B) Know where the fire alarms and extinguishers are located
    (C) Carry as many patient files as you can as you leave the facility
    (D) Shout loudly about what is happening so all patients can hear

11. In case of earthquakes it is best to
    (A) Go outside and find the closest tall building
    (B) Shout if trapped under debris
    (C) Get under a sturdy piece of furniture
    (D) Stand on a piece of tall furniture to get as far away from the ground as possible

12. In case of an active shooter it is best to
    (A) Run outside to find a safe place to hide
    (B) Keep your phone ringer on in case police or family members need to contact you
    (C) Secure the door by moving a heavy piece of furniture in front of it
    (D) Find and confront the shooter

Name: ______________________________

7

Patient Scheduling, Reception, and Related Communication

1. Describe approaches to patient scheduling

True or False

1. ____ MAs do not schedule appointments.
2. ____ Most medical offices use paper appointment books.
3. ____ Practice management systems allow appointment intervals to be blocked off as needed.
4. ____ A patient scheduling a follow-up exam is scheduled for a longer time than a new patient.
5. ____ A medical office's appointment book can be used as evidence in court.

Matching

Match each description to a form of scheduling. Letters may be used more than once.

6. ____ Four people may be scheduled for the same 60-minute period.
7. ____ This is a good match for a practice where patients often arrive either early or late for appointments.
8. ____ Two people are given the same appointment time.
9. ____ A pediatrician seeing sick children only in the mornings is an example.
10. ____ This schedule works best in practices with a large number of patients with urgent needs, such as patients with diabetes.
11. ____ Most medical offices use this method of scheduling.
12. ____ Patients are given appointments based on conditions or illnesses.
13. ____ This is a common form of scheduling in urgent care clinics.
14. ____ Part of the hour may be left open for patients who need to be worked in.
15. ____ Patients do not need an appointment.

(A) Timed

(B) Open hours

(C) Wave

(D) Modified wave

(E) Double-booking

(F) Cluster

2. Explain the process of scheduling a new patient

Fill in the Blank

1. New patients are patients who have never seen the provider or who have not been seen at a practice for ____________________ years or ______________.
2. The MA must get the patient's medical insurance information. This includes information about the ____________________, or the person who holds the insurance.
3. The ____________________________ is an electronic tool used by many facilities to communicate with patients and give them access to their healthcare information.
4. New patients are usually asked to arrive ______________________ early for the first appointment.

3. Explain the process of scheduling returning patients

Short Answer

1. List three things that should be noted in the appointment record for a returning patient.

___

___

___

2. When are returning patient appointments often made?

___

___

3. List three types of appointment reminders that may be used for returning patients.

___

___

___

4. Discuss the management of schedule changes

Multiple Choice

1. What should an MA do if a patient calls with a medical emergency?
   (A) Take notes about the patient's symptoms and show the provider right away
   (B) Transfer the patient's call to the provider right away
   (C) Direct the patient to go to the nearest emergency room
   (D) Tell the patient to hang up and call 911

2. Which of the following is true about MAs and triage?
   (A) Triage is beyond the scope of practice for an MA; MAs do not perform triage.
   (B) MAs can only perform triage when a licensed healthcare provider is not available.
   (C) MAs can perform triage if a provider is present in the facility to supervise.
   (D) MAs can perform triage if a patient's condition is not life-threatening.

3. Patients with urgent needs
   (A) Are usually told to go to an urgent care clinic
   (B) Are usually told to call 911
   (C) Are usually worked in to a provider's schedule the same day
   (D) Are usually scheduled for the first available appointment

4. What should be done when a patient calls a week in advance to cancel an appointment?
   (A) The patient should be asked to find a different provider.
   (B) The patient should be asked to reschedule.
   (C) The patient should be warned that cancelling will delay needed care.
   (D) The patient should be warned that there is still a charge for cancelled appointments.

5. How is a missed appointment often documented in the appointment book and in the patient's record?
   (A) With the initials *NS* for *no-show*
   (B) With the initials *RS* for *reschedule*
   (C) With the word *noncompliant*
   (D) With a red letter X

6. Which type of scheduling can reduce disruptions caused by patients arriving late for appointments?
   (A) Cluster
   (B) Wave
   (C) Open hours
   (D) Timed

7. Which of the following is true of walk-in patients?
   (A) They must be given an appointment for a later date and asked to come back.
   (B) They are always referred to the nearest urgent care clinic.
   (C) The MA performs triage to decide if a walk-in patient needs to be seen that day.
   (D) They may be worked in or seen during time set aside for walk-ins.

8. In what situations should a patient be notified about a delay in seeing the provider?
   (A) If the provider will be more than 5–10 minutes late
   (B) If the provider will be more than 20–30 minutes late
   (C) If the provider will be more than 45 minutes late
   (D) If the provider will be more than an hour late

9. An OB/GYN is called to the hospital to help deliver a baby. She will be more than an hour late for several appointments. What should the MA do?
   (A) Tell the patients the provider is delayed and the office will buy them lunch while they wait.
   (B) Tell the patients they may have to wait a few minutes.
   (C) Tell the patients about the situation and offer to reschedule them for another day.
   (D) Suggest that the patients go home and call later in the day to reschedule.

10. What is the term for a licensed provider who cares for patients temporarily when a provider is away?
   (A) Substitute doctor
   (B) Temp provider
   (C) *Res ipsa loquitur*
   (D) *Locum tenens*

5. Discuss the patient check-in process

True or False

1. ____ Patients must read and sign privacy notifications and consent forms at every visit.

2. ____ The reason for a patient's visit must be written on the sign-in sheet.

3. ____ Patients must give the medical office permission to release information to their insurance company if the office manages insurance claims.

4. ____ Because of HIPAA regulations, sign-in sheets cannot record insurance information.

5. ____ Medical offices never collect payment during check-in.

6. Describe the patient checkout process

Short Answer

1. When does patient checkout happen?

____

____

2. What is given to a patient after any payment is made?

____

____

3. List at least two other items a patient may be given at checkout.

____

____

7. Describe the management of referrals to other medical offices or facilities

Crossword

Across

2. The provider may delegate the MA to provide the patient with this before a test or procedure.
3. After insurance approval is received, this is the next thing the MA does for the appointment.
6. Many insurance companies require this to confirm that a service will be covered.

Down

1. A cardiologist is an example of this type of provider.
4. This is made when a patient needs to see another healthcare provider.
5. Who should clarify any questions the MA cannot answer?

Name: ______________________________

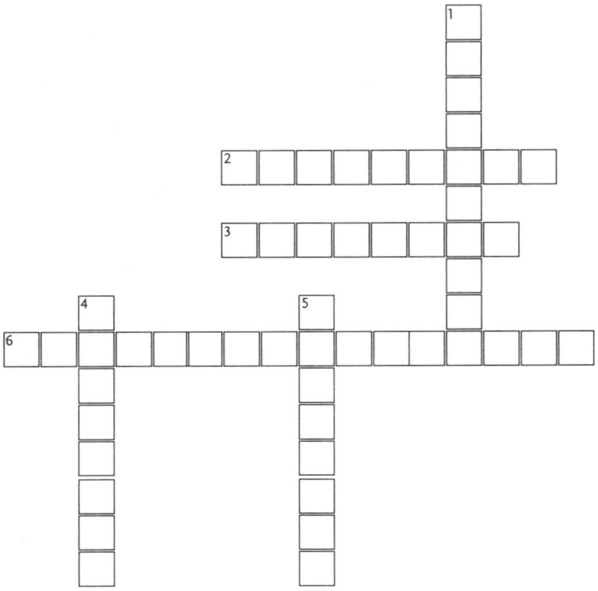

8. List guidelines for communicating with dissatisfied or angry patients

Multiple Choice

1. What communication techniques can help when a patient is dissatisfied?
   (A) Calling in a professional negotiator and documenting everything that is said
   (B) Speaking in a tone that is softer than the patient's and looking down to seem less aggressive
   (C) Cutting the patient off any time they say something untrue and asking them to start over
   (D) Practicing active listening and making eye contact

2. Which of the following is true about patients who are angry or dissatisfied?
   (A) It may result from the patient's anxiety over a medical condition.
   (B) It is usually a result of something the MA did wrong.
   (C) It is best to ignore an angry or dissatisfied patient.
   (D) Angry or dissatisfied patients must be escorted out by security.

Fill in the Blank

3. Being ______________ means that the MA understands the patient's thoughts and feelings.
4. Asking a patient questions allows the MA to ______________ the message and get ______________.
5. The MA should give the patient time to ______________ their thoughts and ______________.
6. The MA should acknowledge the patient's feelings and ______________.

9. Discuss guidelines for written communication

True or False

1. ____ MAs may write letters, emails, or patient portal messages on behalf of the provider.
2. ____ Reference lines are only used in email messages.
3. ____ Communications are filed separately from a patient's medical record.
4. ____ Many medical offices have templates for commonly used documents.

10. Describe the process of legally terminating a provider-patient relationship

Short Answer

1. What can a patient do to terminate her relationship with a provider if she is unsatisfied?

____

____

2. What must a provider do when terminating a relationship with a patient?

____

____

Name: ______________________________

3. What is one reason missed appointments and noncompliance with a treatment plan should be documented carefully in a patient's record?

____

____

4. What are two things that should be included in a termination letter?

____

____

____

____

____

Name: ______________________________

8

Medical Record Management

1. Understand EMR, EHR, and paper filing systems

Short Answer

Read the following and mark EHR *for statements that apply only to electronic health records,* EMR *for statements that apply only to electronic medical records,* P *for statements that apply only to paper records, and* ALL *for statements that apply to all types of records.*

1. ____ Includes provider notes describing assessments, diagnoses, and treatment plans
2. ____ Can only be accessed by a single healthcare facility
3. ____ Requires a large amount of space for storage
4. ____ Must be kept confidential
5. ____ Most traditional organization is by source or category
6. ____ Can be accessed across many healthcare systems
7. ____ CMS provides incentives for meaningful use.
8. ____ Management is a critical responsibility for MAs.

2. Describe patient portals for electronic records access

Multiple Choice

1. What does a patient portal provide?
   (A) An online connection allowing patients to order their own diagnostic tests
   (B) An online connection between the patient and their provider
   (C) An online connection where patients at the same practice can communicate with each other
   (D) An online connection where all providers involved in a patient's care can communicate with each other

2. What types of documents may commonly be sent to a patient using a patient portal?
   (A) A new patient information packet
   (B) A warning about noncompliance
   (C) A termination letter
   (D) A list of other patients who have similar diagnoses and may want to form a support group

3. What is the most common way for a patient to get access to a patient portal?
   (A) Sending a direct message to the MA from any social media application
   (B) Calling the medical office and requesting access
   (C) Using a link in an email sent by the MA
   (D) Filling out a request form with the provider's business office

3. Discuss legal issues related to patient records

Matching

Match each term to a definition below. Use each letter only once.

1. ____ Firewall
2. ____ Magnetic degaussing
3. ____ Cloud-based storage
4. ____ Shredding
5. ____ Encryption

(A) A procedure used to completely erase electronic records

(B) Converting electronic records into codes to prevent unauthorized access

(C) Data storage that is completely online

(D) A security feature that protects computer files from being accessed by or sent to unauthorized users

(E) A method of destroying paper files

Fill in the Blank

6. The ______________________ owns a patient's medical records.
7. Facilities may legally charge patients a fee for creating copies of ______________, but the fee must be ______________.
8. CMS recommends that medical records be kept ______________ or for a minimum of ______________ after the record is closed.

4. Describe scheduling, patient record, and billing software functions

Short Answer

1. List three practice management functions that may be included in EHR software.

____

____

____

2. What is an MA doing when they *index* material in a patient's EHR?

____

____

____

3. What does *CPOE* stand for? List something that may be ordered by CPOE.

____

____

____

4. What does a test order status of *pending* mean?

____

____

____

5. List three ways an EHR or practice management system may send reminder notifications to patients.

____

____

____

6. What are two advantages of sending prescriptions to a pharmacy electronically?

____

____

____

____

____

7. What is listed on a superbill?

____

____

____

____

____

Name: ______________________________

8. List at least three things an MA may print for a patient from an EHR system.

____

____

____

____

____

9. How might the EHR be used for a referral?

____

____

____

____

____

Name: ___________________________________

9

Medical Insurance and Coding

1. Explain the basics of health insurance

Matching

Match each term to a definition below. Use each letter only once.

1. ____ First party
2. ____ Second party
3. ____ Third party
4. ____ Claim
5. ____ Premium
6. ____ Copayment
7. ____ Policy
8. ____ Benefits
9. ____ Coinsurance
10. ____ Out-of-pocket maximum
11. ____ Deductible
12. ____ Guarantor
13. ____ Dependent

(A) The person financially responsible for paying a medical bill

(B) The services covered (paid for) by an insurance policy and how much may be paid for each service

(C) A payment made by a patient based on a percentage of healthcare costs

(D) A request to an insurance company for payment

(E) The patient

(F) The product offered by an insurance company

(G) The amount that must be paid for services by the subscriber before an insurer will pay any healthcare costs

(H) The highest amount a subscriber will pay before an insurer pays 100% of healthcare costs

(I) The health insurance company that pays for services

(J) Family members of a subscriber to a health insurance policy who are also covered by the policy

(K) Monthly payments to an insurance company; required to maintain eligibility

(L) The provider

(M) A set amount (e.g., $25) that must be paid by a patient for a visit/service

Fill in the Blank

14. A summary of coverage provided to a patient by an insurance company after a claim is made is called a(n) ______________________________________.

15. A summary of coverage provided to a provider by an insurance company after a claim is made is called a(n) ______________________________________.

16. ______________________ services are those services essential to the patient's health and well-being.

17. The standard fee set by a health insurance company for a specific healthcare service is the ______________________.

18. If the provider is part of an insurer's network, any amount the provider charges above the insurer's allowable amount must be ______________________.

Name: ______________________________

2. Discuss private insurance programs

Crossword

Across

3. Under an indemnity plan, what a provider's charges must be considered to be, in addition to customary and reasonable
5. The type of flat fee an HMO may pay a provider for each patient
7. Point-of-service plans have lower premiums and copayments than other types of managed care plans, but these may be larger.
10. The type of provider organization in which members are encouraged, but not required, to see providers in the insurance company's network

Down

1. The type of provider organization in which members do not usually need to have a PCP or get referrals for specialists, but they may only see network providers for routine care
2. In managed care, what a PCP is often called due to their role managing access to all healthcare services a patient receives
4. The name of the insurance-purchasing forum made possible by the ACA and offered on the website healthcare.gov
6. Something added to an insurance policy that changes the terms of the policy
8. Private health insurance plans are purchased through this or by an individual.
9. Workers who lose group insurance may use this program to purchase the same insurance privately for a certain period of time.

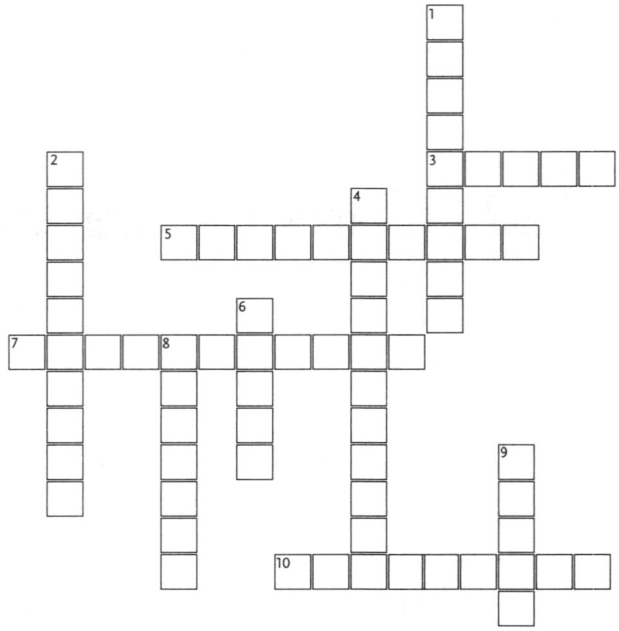

3. Describe government-funded insurance programs

Multiple Choice

1. In addition to covering people 65 and older, Medicare covers
   (A) People with a low income
   (B) People who live in certain states or territories
   (C) All military veterans
   (D) People with end-stage kidney disease
2. Medicaid is administered and operated
   (A) At the state level
   (B) By individual medical facilities
   (C) By Medicare Administrative Contractors
   (D) At the county level
3. Medicare Part C
   (A) Is required and covers prescription drugs
   (B) Is optional and offers benefits to replace Parts A and B
   (C) Is also called *Medigap*
   (D) Usually has very high premiums

4. Medicare's Accountable Care Organization (ACO) model has the goal of
   (A) Cutting costs by reducing the number of services elderly patients receive
   (B) Ensuring that all providers offer exactly the same care to all Medicare patients
   (C) Having providers work together to give elderly patients high-quality care at a lower cost
   (D) Paying only for treatments the ACO is sure will be successful

5. Which part of Medicare covers outpatient office visits and supplies?
   (A) Part A
   (B) Part B
   (C) Part C
   (D) Part D

6. What program provides low-cost health insurance for children in families that have lower incomes but earn too much to qualify for Medicaid?
   (A) IHS
   (B) CHIP
   (C) TRICARE
   (D) CHAMPVA

7. Which of the following is true about the Indian Health Service?
   (A) It is an insurance program for American Indians and Alaska Natives.
   (B) It is not an insurance program but it makes insurance unnecessary.
   (C) People who receive health care through Indian Health Service may qualify for Medicare, Medicaid, and other federal programs.
   (D) Indian Health Service care and programs are available to all US citizens.

8. Dependents of military veterans who were disabled or killed in the line of duty are covered by
   (A) TRICARE Select
   (B) CHAMPVA
   (C) CHIP
   (D) TRICARE for Life

9. Which of these health insurance programs could cover a 21-year-old college student who is the unmarried dependent of an active duty member of the US military?
   (A) CHIP
   (B) TRICARE Reserve Select
   (C) TRICARE Young Adult
   (D) TRICARE Select

10. If an established patient is seen for care related to a workers' compensation claim, what is done to protect against unnecessary release of PHI?
    (A) The patient is asked not to tell their employer that their usual doctor is managing the workers' compensation care.
    (B) The patient must sign a form saying they will not discuss care related to the claim at work.
    (C) Records related to the workers' compensation claim are kept separate from the rest of the patient's medical record.
    (D) A separate tab is created in the patient's file to document care related to the workers' compensation claim.

4. Explain coordination of benefits

Fill in the Blank

1. When a patient is covered by more than one insurance policy, one policy is considered the ______________________________ and the other is the ______________________________.

2. If a child is covered by policies held by both parents, the ____________________ rule is often used to determine which parent's insurance is primary.

3. Under this rule, the policy of the parent with the ______________________________ in the year is the primary insurance for the child.

4. ____________________ plans have detailed COB rules. MAs should check the plans in question to determine which program pays ____________________.

5. Describe the insurance claims process

Short Answer

1. What does NPI stand for? What is it?

____

____

____

____

2. What form must a patient sign to give their insurance company permission to make payments directly to the medical office?

____

____

3. How often does a patient need to sign a release of information form giving a medical office permission to share PHI with their insurance company?

____

4. When should insurance claims be submitted?

____

____

5. What form is the standard insurance form used for paper billing?

____

6. Which type of claim usually takes longer to pay: a claim filed electronically or a claim filed on paper?

____

____

7. What does a clearinghouse do?

____

____

____

____

____

____

True or False

8. ____ When a provider's office sends claims electronically to the insurance company it is called *direct billing*.

9. ____ Most insurance companies have a time limit for filing claims.

10. ____ An insurance claim must include information about the location where the service was provided.

11. ____ Insurance companies do not consider whether a medical service provided is appropriate for the patient's diagnosis.

12. ____ A *clean claim* is one that is accepted by the insurance company for payment.

13. ____ A claim that is rejected due to errors can be corrected and resubmitted.

6. Discuss the need for preauthorization for certain medical treatments

Matching

Use each letter only once.

1. ____ Patient's insurance card
2. ____ Advance Beneficiary Notice (ABN)
3. ____ Preauthorization number
4. ____ Precertification
5. ____ Preauthorization
6. ____ Appeal

(A) The approval of a procedure as medically necessary by a patient's insurance company

(B) One place an MA can look for information about services that require preauthorization

(C) Medicare form informing a patient that a service will not be covered

(D) Must be on the patient's claim form when billing for a service that requires preauthorization

(E) Confirmation that a patient's insurance policy covers a particular procedure

(F) Usually requires additional proof that a planned procedure is medically necessary

7. Understand the purpose of medical coding systems

Multiple Choice

1. What were medical coding systems first developed to track?
   (A) The average amounts of insurance payments for different treatments
   (B) The most commonly prescribed medications
   (C) Information about morbidity (disease) and mortality (death)
   (D) The number of providers in a geographic area

2. The system that was originally called the International Statistical Classification of Diseases, Injuries and Causes of Death is now called the ICD. What does *ICD* stand for?
   (A) The International Classification of Diseases
   (B) The International Cause of Death list
   (C) The Injury Cause Definition
   (D) The Internal Classification for Doctors

3. The CDC developed a clinical version of the ICD that is used for
   (A) Tracking deaths
   (B) Tracking disease trends and epidemics around the world
   (C) Describing outpatient treatments
   (D) Diagnosis coding

8. Discuss the ICD coding system

Matching

Use each letter only once.

1. ____ Encounter
2. ____ Billable code
3. ____ Diagnosis category
4. ____ ICD-CM
5. ____ ICD-PCS
6. ____ The letter *Z*
7. ____ Conventions
8. ____ The letter *X*

(A) System used to code most inpatient procedures
(B) Used as a placeholder in ICD-10-CM codes
(C) The general rules for using ICD and other coding systems
(D) The first three characters (one letter and two numbers) in an ICD-10-CM code
(E) Used as a placeholder in ICD-10-PCS codes
(F) A code that can be used to support an insurance claim
(G) System used to communicate information about diagnoses
(H) Term for a healthcare service provided

Fill in the Blank

9. When using the ICD-CM, it is important to choose the most ______________ code possible to describe the patient's ______________.

10. At least one ICD-10-PCS code is used for every ______________ procedure performed.

11. The ICD-CM is organized into a(n) ______________ Index and a(n) ______________ List.

9. Discuss the CPT coding system

True or False

1. ____ *CPT* stands for *Clinical Patient Therapies.*
2. ____ The CPT Tabular List contains codes in six sections.
3. ____ The CDC developed the CPT coding system to bill for outpatient procedures.
4. ____ There is a category of CPT codes used to track performance and quality.
5. ____ Evaluation and management (E/M) codes are used for most patient visits.
6. ____ One of the factors that determines the correct E/M code for a visit is whether a patient is new or established.

7. ____ A bundled code is one that describes all the procedures done for a single patient over a one-month period.

8. ____ Category I CPT codes are used for billing and are always numeric.

10. Discuss the HCPCS coding system

Short Answer

1. List four things covered by HCPCS codes.

____

____

____

____

2. What is one example of a modifier that may be used with an HCPCS code?

____

____

____

3. What letter begins all codes for ambulance and transportation services?

____

4. If a patient is seen at a medical office for a wound dressing change, what may be billed using an HCPCS code?

____

____

11. Discuss the importance of accuracy in coding

Multiple Choice

1. What happens when an insurance company *downcodes* a claim for reimbursement?
   (A) The medical office is paid more than the claim requested.
   (B) The medical office is paid less than the claim requested.
   (C) The claim is rejected for payment.
   (D) The claim is sent to a clearinghouse for review.

2. If a medical office intentionally submits separate claims for services that have a bundled code, they are guilty of
   (A) A mistake
   (B) An audit
   (C) Abuse
   (D) Larceny

3. Submitting a claim for a higher level of service than what was provided is called
   (A) Upcoding
   (B) Downcoding
   (C) Overcoding
   (D) Undercoding

4. A clean claim shows a clear code linkage between
   (A) Goods and services
   (B) Diagnosis and procedures
   (C) Cause and effect
   (D) Treatment and results

5. A review of medical records to make sure proper billing guidelines are followed is called a(n)
   (A) Evaluation
   (B) Investigation
   (C) Code check
   (D) Audit

6. Which of the following is an example of fraud?
   (A) A medical office regularly bills insurance companies for services that were not performed.
   (B) A medical office uses bundled codes any time they are required.
   (C) A medical office requests that patients pay in full at the time of a visit.
   (D) A new MA accidentally submits separate codes for procedures that have a bundled code available.

10

Billing, Collections, and Accounting

1. Discuss physician fees and patient billing

Matching

Use each letter only once.

1. ____ Sliding scale
2. ____ Billing cycle
3. ____ Credit
4. ____ Debit
5. ____ Ledger
6. ____ Physician fee schedule

(A) A record of all financial transactions

(B) A list of the cost of services provided by licensed healthcare professionals

(C) Created to collect outstanding balances; usually involves grouping patients alphabetically or by date of service

(D) A set system for adjusting customary fees for patients with low incomes

(E) Business expenses

(F) Business income

Short Answer

7. List four examples of expenses a medical practice may have.

____

____

____

____

____

8. What is created at every patient visit and lists diagnosis and procedure codes along with any charges?

____

9. What could happen if a medical office gives discounted services to some patients and not to others?

____

____

10. What is the legal term for a person who lives in extreme poverty? What should an MA keep to help support patients in this situation?

____

____

____

____

11. After an insurance company has made its payment and the patient has paid the required copayment or coinsurance amount, what should the patient account show?

____

____

12. How should a medical practice manage discounts such as cash discounts for uninsured patients or professional courtesy discounts for other healthcare providers or staff members?

____

____

____

____

Name: ______________________________

2. Describe patient accounts and statements

Fill in the Blank

1. Schedule a regular ____________________ ____________________ to perform accounting tasks.
2. Calculation errors are ____________________ in an electronic system, but when numbers are entered ____________________, the calculations will not be correct.
3. Organize manual financial records ____________________.
4. Records must be kept a minimum of ____________________ years after a tax return has been filed for a particular year.
5. Patients with outstanding balances are billed ____________________.
6. If a patient's insurance allows $100 for a procedure that normally costs $125, the MA records a(n) __________ discount to the patient's balance.
7. A(n) ____________________ is a bank draft that directs funds to be taken from a bank account to pay an expense.
8. Checks may be returned to the practice for ______________________________ if there is not enough money in the patient's ______________________________ to cover the amount of the check.
9. The practice pays ____________________ for each debit or credit card transaction.
10. ____________________ is money that is paid at a set percentage rate for a debt.
11. The federal Truth in Lending Act (TILA) requires that patients be told the ____________________ of payment plans, including any ____________________. They must also be told in advance about payment due dates and ____________________.

3. Understand the collection process and the life cycle of a patient bill

Multiple Choice

1. What does an aging report show?
   (A) Patient demographic information sorted by age
   (B) The length of time that has passed since a charge was posted to an account
   (C) The length of time a practice has accepted a particular type of insurance
   (D) The success of patient treatments sorted by patient age
2. When a patient account has a payment that is more than 120 days past due it is usually considered
   (A) A total loss
   (B) Criminally overdue
   (C) Delinquent
   (D) Written off
3. What regulations should a medical office follow to collect a past due balance ethically?
   (A) The Truth in Lending Act (TILA)
   (B) The Patient Protection and Affordable Care Act (ACA)
   (C) The Healthcare Quality Improvement Act (HCQIA)
   (D) The Fair Debt Collection Practices Act (FDCPA)
4. When is a patient debt usually considered uncollectible?
   (A) After three letters have been sent with no response
   (B) After 60 days
   (C) After the patient has not returned three messages left by phone
   (D) After a patient's check has bounced
5. How are collection agencies paid for their services?
   (A) They receive a flat fee for every debt turned over to them.
   (B) They charge a monthly fee to collect as many debts as a practice needs collected.
   (C) They keep a percentage of the debt they collect.
   (D) They collect more than what is owed to the provider and keep the extra.

Short Answer

Use numbers 1–11 to order the following steps in the life cycle of a patient bill.

6. ____ If payment is not made, a second bill is sent.
7. ____ A claim is made with the patient's insurance company for the remaining amount.
8. ____ The patient sees their provider and pays their copay at the time of the visit.
9. ____ The patient is billed for any remaining balance for which they are responsible.
10. ____ If the balance remains unpaid, the practice may choose to send a certified letter of termination to the patient and send the account to collections.
11. ____ Immediately following the encounter, the MA records the cost of the service in the patient's account.
12. ____ After the second billing cycle, the MA should contact the patient to ask about the balance and request payment.
13. ____ The amount paid in copayment/coinsurance is credited against the total cost (subtracted from the amount due).
14. ____ The insurer processes the claim and sends payment and RA to the provider.
15. ____ If the balance is not paid by the third billing cycle, that bill may include a warning that it will be submitted to a collection agency.
16. ____ The MA records the insurer's payment in the patient's account along with any charge adjustments shown on the RA statement.

4. Explain accounts payable and receivable and practice assets and liabilities

True or False

1. ____ A monthly bill from a company that manages biohazardous waste for a medical office is an example of an account payable.
2. ____ In order for a business to be successful, accounts payable should be a larger amount than accounts receivable.
3. ____ Expected payments from insurance companies are an example of accounts receivable.
4. ____ *Assets* and *liabilities* are different words for the same thing.
5. ____ A practice's net worth is calculated by subtracting the practice's liabilities from its assets.
6. ____ Accounts receivable are counted as part of a practice's assets.

5. Discuss bank accounts and check handling

Crossword

Across

3. The manual or electronic record of all debits and credits to a bank account; may use a one-line or two-line system
4. The person who receives payment from a check
6. Separation of duties protects against this type of theft, in which an employee steals from their employer.
7. A number that is unique to a bank and is printed on a check along with the account number

Name: ______________________________

Down

1. The term used to describe a check that has the proper elements to be payable
2. The signing or stamping of the back of a check
5. This type of bank account is used for daily financial transactions.

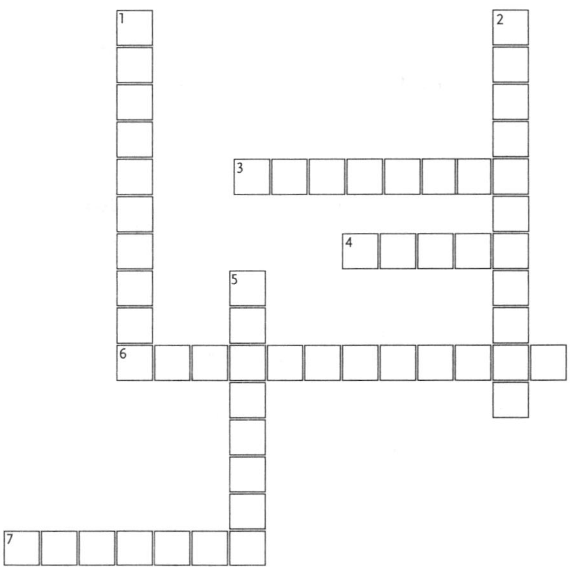

6. Describe supply purchasing and the management of petty cash

Short Answer

1. How is a blanket purchase order used?

____

____

____

____

____

2. What does *consumable* mean?

____

____

3. What are consumable items called?

____

4. What is the benefit of being part of a purchasing group?

____

____

5. How soon should an invoice be paid in order to remain in good standing with a vendor?

____

6. What is written on the payee line of a check used to get petty cash?

____

7. After a shipment of supplies arrives at a medical office, what must be done with the packing slip?

____

____

____

____

11

Office Equipment and Supplies

1. Describe computer hardware and associated equipment

Matching

Match each item to the correct category of equipment. Letters may be used more than once.

1. ____ Modems, routers, and switches are examples.
2. ____ May be used to allow patients to complete and sign paperless forms during check-in
3. ____ Often not thought of as computers but can perform many computing tasks
4. ____ Sometimes mounted on carts that can be moved from room to room and used to track patient care
5. ____ Make it possible for devices to share access to the same hardware, data, and/or services
6. ____ Self-contained units with a screen, keyboard, and input device
7. ____ May include a webcam and a microphone or headset
8. ____ Small, portable external ones require special care for confidentiality.
9. ____ Their portability makes them easy to use when documenting patient care.
10. ____ One part may be called a "tower."

(A) Desktop computers

(B) Laptop or notebook computers

(C) Tablet computers

(D) Smartphones

(E) Equipment for telehealth visits

(F) Storage devices

(G) Networking hardware

Multiple Choice

11. What type of software are EHR systems?
    (A) Word processing
    (B) Internet browser
    (C) Spreadsheet
    (D) Database

12. What is the difference between software and hardware?
    (A) Software is used on portable devices and hardware is used on desktop devices.
    (B) Software is a program run by a computer and hardware is the computer and computer equipment.
    (C) Software is the computer and computer equipment and hardware is a program run by a computer.
    (D) Software is a computer that is not secured for confidentiality and hardware is a computer that is properly secured.

13. An internal file-sharing system that can only be used by computers on an office network is called
    (A) The internet
    (B) A database
    (C) An intranet
    (D) An IT hub

14. What small device may be used to provide backup power to machines and devices in case of a power failure?
    (A) A surge protector
    (B) An uninterruptible power supply (UPS)
    (C) A signal switch
    (D) A generator

2. Discuss other common office equipment

Short Answer

1. List four possible functions of a multifunction office copier.

______

______

______

______

2. Why might a medical office have a calculator or adding machine?

______

______

______

3. List three types of safety and security equipment common in a medical office.

______

______

______

4. How do documents containing PHI have to be shredded?

______

______

______

______

______

5. What are three common options on a medical office's telephone answering system?

______

______

______

______

6. List five tasks an MA may be assigned to open a medical office for the day.

______

______

______

______

______

______

______

7. List four tasks an MA may be assigned to close a medical office for the day.

______

______

______

______

______

______

3. Understand equipment maintenance

True or False

1. ____ MAs need to know how to service each type of equipment in the office or facility where they work.
2. ____ When equipment is leased, the vendor usually maintains it.
3. ____ Equipment plugged into a surge protector or UPS should be unplugged as part of closing the office each day.
4. ____ Computer viruses damage computer hardware.
5. ____ Keeping the office tidy is the main reason to remove dust from office machines.
6. ____ Spilling a cup of soda on office equipment can cause permanent damage.

7. ____ Turning off the power strip where a desktop computer is plugged in is the best way to shut down the computer for the night.

8. ____ If an MA cannot find a paper manual for office equipment, they will probably have to call the manufacturer and order a replacement manual.

Multiple Choice

9. Where do offices commonly keep information about equipment maintenance?
   (A) In the EHR database
   (B) On maintenance log sheets
   (C) On the user portal of each manufacturer's website
   (D) On a sticky note attached to each piece of equipment

10. What is the first step in basic troubleshooting?
   (A) Call the service number listed in the instruction manual.
   (B) Call a local technician authorized by the manufacturer.
   (C) Check to be sure that the machine is plugged in and turned on.
   (D) Ask the provider to check the equipment.

4. Discuss office and medical supplies inventory

Short Answer

1. What information is usually included in an equipment inventory?

____

____

____

____

____

____

2. List ten common clinical supplies used in a medical office.

____

____

____

____

____

____

____

____

3. List ten common administrative supplies used in a medical office.

____

____

____

____

____

____

____

____

4. List five common general supplies used in a medical office.

____

____

____

____

____

____

Fill in the Blank

5. An organized system for ____________________ makes tracking supply ____________________ more efficient.

Name: ______________________________

6. All supplies of one kind should be stored ____________________.

7. Supplies are rotated for storage so that the ____________________ supplies are used first. This is important because many supplies have ____________________.

8. MAs should know the ____________________ for each supply. This is the time that an item should be ordered.

9. A(n) ____________________ is the amount of an item that should be kept in case there is a shipping delay or the item is out of stock.

10. The formula for calculating the reorder point for a supply is (amount of the item that is used ____________________ x turnaround time from ____________________ to delivery) + a safety stock.

Short Answer

For each of the following situations, answer the questions to calculate the reorder point for the supply. Remember that this is the formula for finding a reorder point:

Amount used per day x days from order to delivery + safety stock = reorder point

11. Hartman Physicians' Group uses an average of 10 lavender-topped blood collection tubes each day. It is currently taking 15 business days for new shipments to arrive. The safety stock is a 3-week supply.

    How many tubes are used each day? _____

    How many days does it take to get a new shipment? _____

    How many tubes are in the safety stock? _____

    The office should reorder when _____ tubes are left.

12. An endocrinology office uses an average of 20 lancets per day. They come in boxes of 100. From order to delivery, reordering takes 1 week. Safety stock is 2 boxes of lancets. What is the reorder point for lancet **boxes**?

    How many boxes of lancets are used each day? (This can be shown as a fraction or decimal.) _____

    How many days does it take to get a new shipment? (Count business days only.) _____

    How many boxes are in the safety stock? _____

    The office should reorder when _____ boxes are left.

13. Exam table paper rolls come in boxes with 12 rolls. Each roll usually lasts through 20 changes. Dr. Letizia is the only provider in her office. On most days she sees 20 patients. It takes 10 business days to receive a new order of exam table paper. Safety stock for this item is 1 box. What is the reorder point?

    How many boxes are used each day? (This can be shown as a fraction or decimal.) _____

    How many days does it take to get a new shipment? _____

    How many boxes are in the safety stock? _____

    The office should reorder when _____ boxes are left. (Round to the nearest whole box.)

12

Introduction to Medical Terminology and Body Systems

1. Understand how to use medical terminology

Multiple Choice

1. With whom should an MA use medical terminology?
   (A) With patients
   (B) With patient family members
   (C) With other care team members
   (D) With the office's business manager

2. Why is it helpful for an MA to use medical terms when describing a patient's signs and symptoms to a provider?
   (A) It is like a secret language that makes it more difficult for the patient to understand.
   (B) It makes the best use of the MA's and the provider's training.
   (C) It makes communication more specific and accurate.
   (D) It shows the provider that the MA is intelligent.

2. Identify common roots, prefixes, and suffixes

Fill in the Blank

1. A(n) __________ is the part of a word that contains its basic meaning or definition.

2. The __________ is the word part that precedes (comes before) the root to help form a new word.

3. The __________ is the word part added to the end of a root that helps form a new word.

4. Word roots in medical terms usually refer to a(n) __________.

5. Prefixes in medical terms usually describe a(n) __________, amount, direction, or time.

6. Suffixes in medical terms usually relate to a(n) __________, disease, or procedure.

7. Combining vowels may be placed between elements in a medical term to make the term __________.

Short Answer

Use the numbers 1–4 to correctly order the steps for defining medical terms.

8. ____ Read the term from right to left.
9. ____ Identify the word root or roots.
10. ____ When in doubt, use a medical dictionary or the resource used at your facility.
11. ____ Identify any prefixes and suffixes contained in the term.

3. Identify common abbreviations

Matching

For each of the following abbreviations, write the letter of the correct term from the list below. Use each letter only once.

1. ____ ac, a.c.
2. ____ amb
3. ____ BM
4. ____ C
5. ____ c/o

Name: ____________

6. ____ CPR
7. ____ F
8. ____ CHF
9. ____ GI
10. ____ DX, dx
11. ____ NKDA
12. ____ NPO
13. ____ TPR
14. ____ pc, p.c.
15. ____ prn, PRN
16. ____ PWB
17. ____ ROM
18. ____ SOB
19. ____ v.s., VS
20. ____ w/c, W/C

(A) Fahrenheit
(B) Gastrointestinal
(C) After meals
(D) Nothing by mouth
(E) Bowel movement
(F) Cardiopulmonary resuscitation
(G) Complains of
(H) Range of motion
(I) Partial weight-bearing
(J) Vital signs
(K) Shortness of breath
(L) Before meals
(M) Congestive heart failure
(N) Wheelchair
(O) As necessary
(P) No known drug allergies
(Q) Celsius
(R) Temperature, pulse, and respirations
(S) Diagnosis
(T) Ambulate, ambulatory

4. Describe anatomical terms of location and direction

Labeling

Write the correct anatomical term of direction on each line in the figures below.

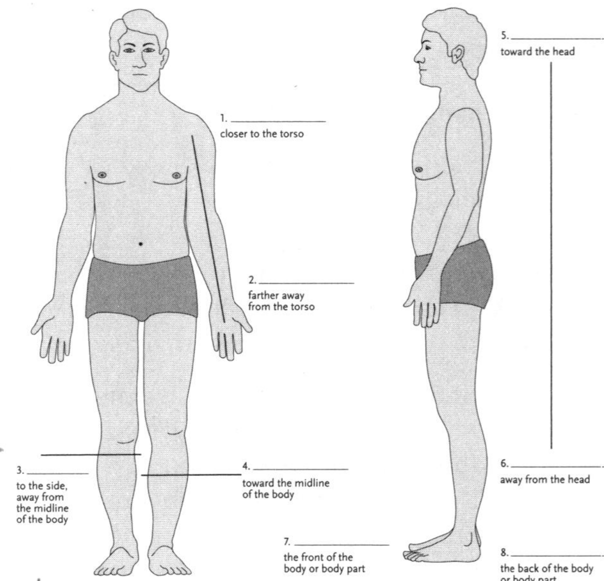

Matching

Match each plane to its definition. Use each letter only once.

9. ____ Coronal/frontal plane
10. ____ Midsagittal/median plane
11. ____ Transverse/axial plane

(A) A plane that divides the body into equal left and right sections
(B) A plane that divides the body into front and back sections
(C) A plane that divides the body into upper and lower sections

Short Answer

Use the blank space after each item below to write the name of the body cavity where it is located.

12. The heart and lungs: ____________
13. The brain: ____________

14. The stomach: ______________________
15. The eyes: ______________________
16. The spinal cord: ______________________
17. The teeth and tongue: ______________________
18. The reproductive organs: ______________________

Labeling

On the numbered blanks, write the name of each region.

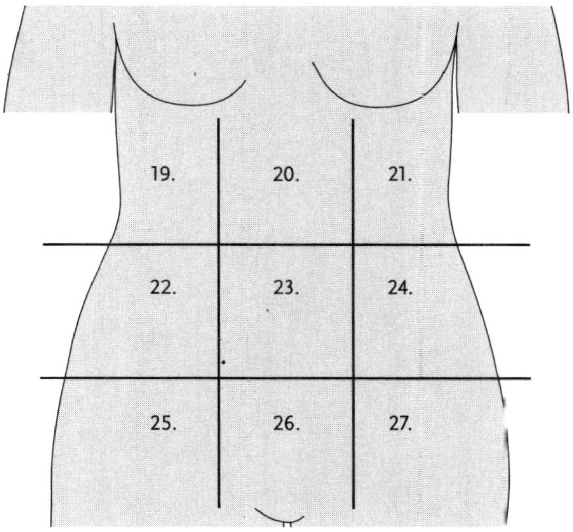

19. ______________________
20. ______________________
21. ______________________
22. ______________________
23. ______________________
24. ______________________
25. ______________________
26. ______________________
27. ______________________

Short Answer

28. List three organs or parts of organs in the right upper quadrant of the abdomen.

____
____
____

29. List four organs or parts of organs in the left upper quadrant of the abdomen.

____
____
____
____

30. List three organs or parts of organs in the right lower quadrant of the abdomen.

____
____
____

31. List three organs or parts of organs in the left lower quadrant of the abdomen.

____
____
____
____

5. Discuss cells, tissues, organs, and body systems

Matching

Match each term to a definition or description below. Use each letter only once.

1. ____ Anatomy
2. ____ Physiology
3. ____ Cells
4. ____ Organs
5. ____ Homeostasis
6. ____ Chromosomes
7. ____ Genes
8. ____ Epithelial tissue
9. ____ Nerve tissue
10. ____ Muscle tissue
11. ____ Connective tissue

Name: ______________________________

(A) Made up of strands of material called DNA; humans receive 23 from each parent

(B) Can contract and relax

(C) The basic units of the body

(D) Forms the skin and linings of the body

(E) A state of balance and stability

(F) Gives humans the ability to respond to their environment

(G) Relates to the structure of body parts

(H) Organized groups of tissues with specific functions

(I) Blood is one form

(J) Relates to body functions

(K) Determine a person's traits

Short Answer

For each of the following items, write the name of the body system described in the space provided.

12. Produces the cells needed to create new human life: ______________________

13. Transports oxygen and nutrients to the cells and removes wastes: ______________________

14. Produces hormones that are secreted in the body: ______________________

15. Breaks down food to supply nutrients to the body's cells: ______________________

16. Protects the body from infection and fluid loss: ______________________

17. Removes wastes and maintains fluid balance: ______________________

18. Supplies oxygen and removes carbon dioxide: ______________________

19. Produces substances that protect the body from disease: ______________________

20. The control center for the body: ______________________

21. Supports the body and gives it the ability to move: ______________________

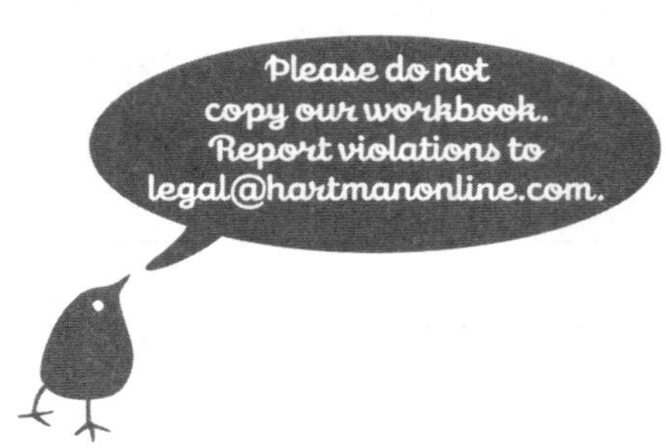

13

Basic Clinical Skills

1. Describe the preparation of the examination room and equipment

Crossword

Across

6. Makes it possible to hear sounds inside the body, such as heart, lung, and abdominal sounds
7. Device used to measure blood pressure
8. The ears are examined with this instrument.
10. This category of medical instrument must be disinfected between patients.
11. This type of instrument is used to widen a body opening for easier inspection.

Down

1. This type of mirror is used to view the interior of the mouth and throat.
2. These protect patient privacy during exams.
3. An instrument used to examine the eyes
4. Measures body temperature
5. These are used to test hearing.
9. This kind of hammer is also called a *percussion hammer.*

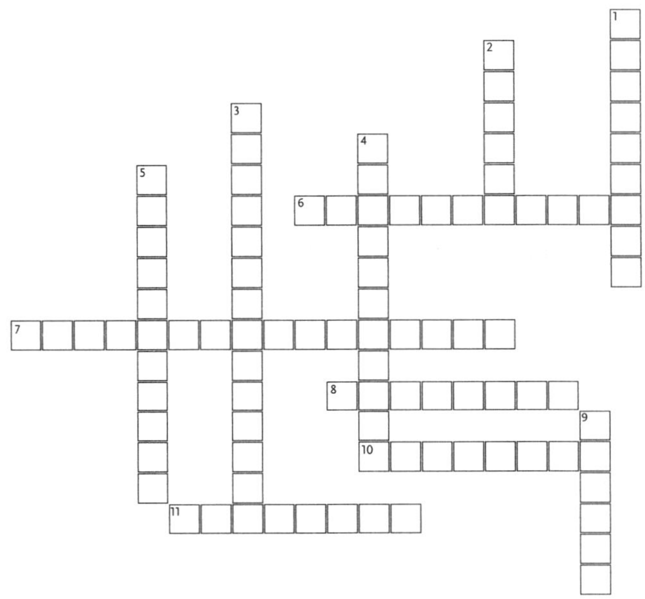

2. List forms of examination

Short Answer

1. List five examples of things a medical assistant could learn about a patient by observation.

____

____

____

____

____

2. List four things that can be examined or found by palpation.

____

____

____

____

3. How does an MA use auscultation during a patient exam? List two examples. How does a provider use auscultation during an exam? List two examples.

____
____
____
____
____
____
____
____

4. Write a brief list of the steps to using a stethoscope correctly.

____
____
____
____
____
____

5. What examination technique involves moving a body part to gather information?

____
____
____

6. What are three things a provider can detect using percussion?

____
____
____
____
____

7. Why might a measuring tape be used during an examination?

____
____
____
____

3. Discuss documentation and professional communication among the healthcare team

Matching

Match each of the Six Cs of Charting to the correct statement below. Use each letter only once.

1. ____ Client's words
2. ____ Clarity
3. ____ Conciseness
4. ____ Completeness
5. ____ Confidentiality
6. ____ Chronological order

(A) All of the information about an encounter should be documented.

(B) Documentation should present a clear picture of what occurred.

(C) Information in the patient's health record should only be discussed with members of the care team.

(D) Quotation marks are used to indicate what the patient said.

(E) MAs should use as few words as possible; abbreviations can help.

(F) This makes the patient's health status and progress easier to understand.

4. Describe patient intake

Multiple Choice

1. Which of the following is true about MAs and patient medications?
   (A) MAs should ask about all prescription medications the patient is taking.
   (B) MAs should ask about all prescription and OTC medications the patient is taking and should also ask about supplements and herbal medicines.
   (C) It is beyond an MA's scope of practice to ask about medications of any kind.
   (D) The MA only needs to ask if any other provider has prescribed a new medication for the patient.

2. Anthropometric measurements include
   (A) Temperature, pulse, and respirations
   (B) All vital signs
   (C) Health conditions of the patient's close relatives
   (D) Body measurements such as height and weight

3. A patient reports that she drinks 3–4 beers per week. This is documented as part of her
   (A) Medical history
   (B) Social history
   (C) Family history
   (D) Medication review

4. A patient reports that he had a hernia repaired 4 years ago. This is documented as part of his
   (A) Medical history
   (B) Social history
   (C) Family history
   (D) Medication review

5. A patient reports that their father died of a stroke at age 58. This is documented as part of their
   (A) Medical history
   (B) Social history
   (C) Family history
   (D) Medication review

6. During intake, a patient reports that he has been having heartburn often over the last month. He had not had problems with heartburn before. It is especially bad if he eats a large meal and gets worse when he lies down. He reports taking TUMS when he has heartburn but says it does not really help. This is the patient's
   (A) Medical history
   (B) Chief complaint
   (C) History of present illness
   (D) Condition summary

7. Which of the following could be an example of a chief complaint?
   (A) Patient reports increased migraine activity
   (B) Patient had open heart surgery 10 years ago
   (C) Patient reports a new medication is working well
   (D) Patient reports that her mother was just diagnosed with breast cancer at age 67

5. Explain the importance of monitoring vital signs

Short Answer

1. What does the term *baseline vital signs* mean?

____

____

____

2. What should an MA do if a patient's vital signs are in the *critical value* category?

____

____

____

3. Why are accurate vital sign measurements important to the provider?

____

____

____

Name: ______________________________

4. List four factors that may affect a patient's vital sign measurements.

____

____

____

____

6. List guidelines for measuring body temperature and observing skin condition

Short Answer

1. What are five sites for measuring body temperature?

____

____

____

____

2. Name seven conditions that indicate a person's temperature should not be taken orally.

____

____

____

____

____

____

____

Labeling

For each of the illustrations of thermometers shown below, write the temperature reading to the nearest tenth degree in the blank provided.

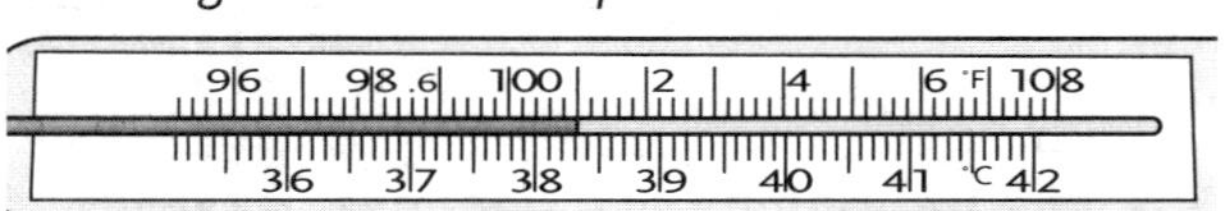

3. ______________________________

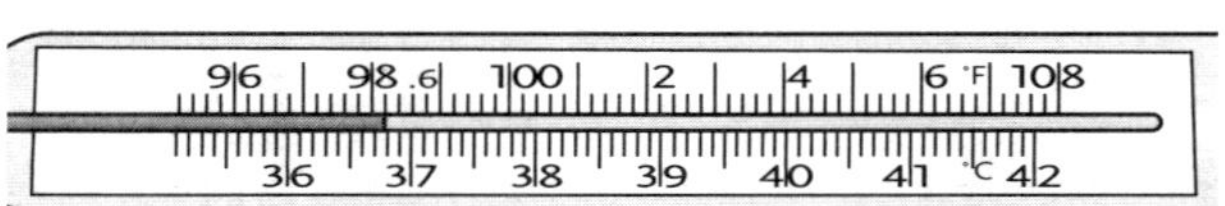

4. ______________________________

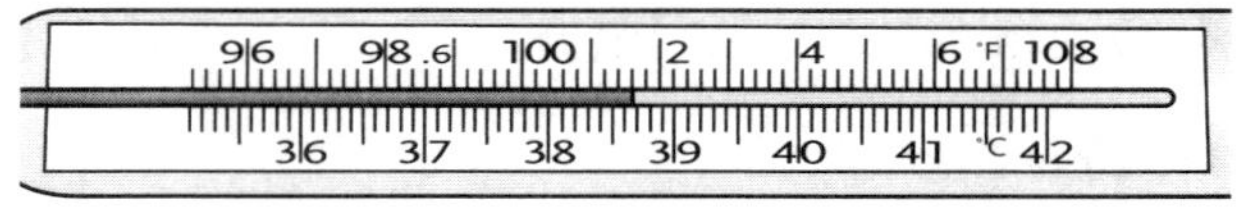

5. ______________________________

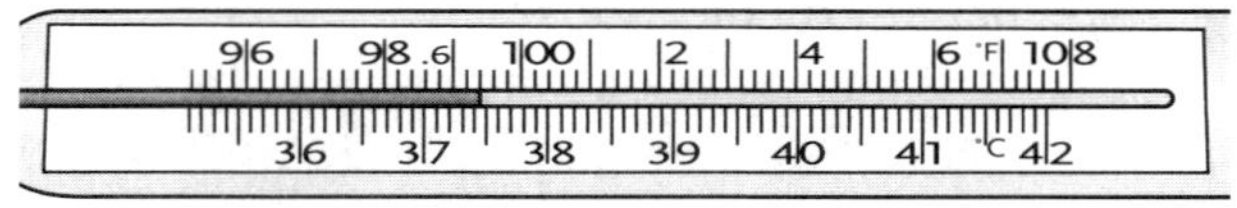

6. ______________________________

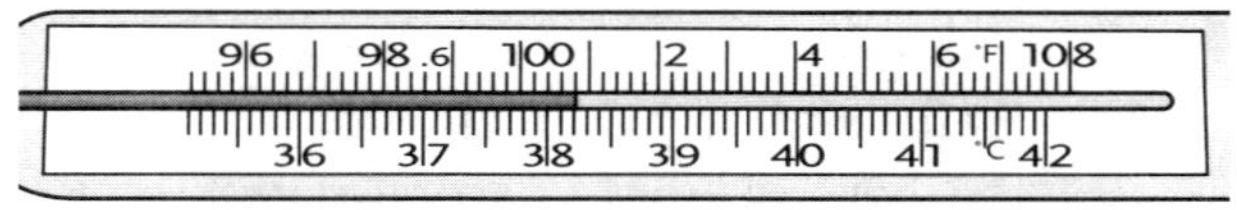

7. ______________________________

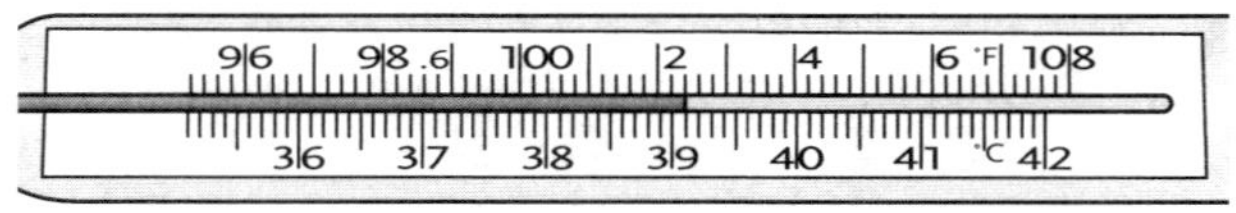

8. ______________________________

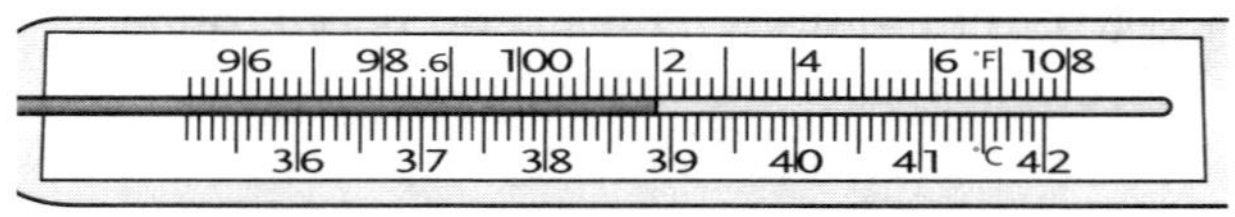

9. ______________________________

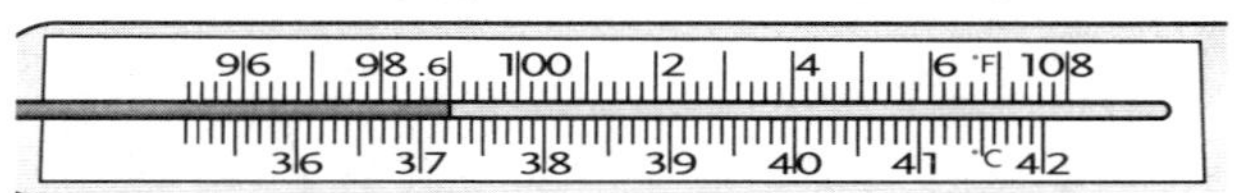

10. ______________________________

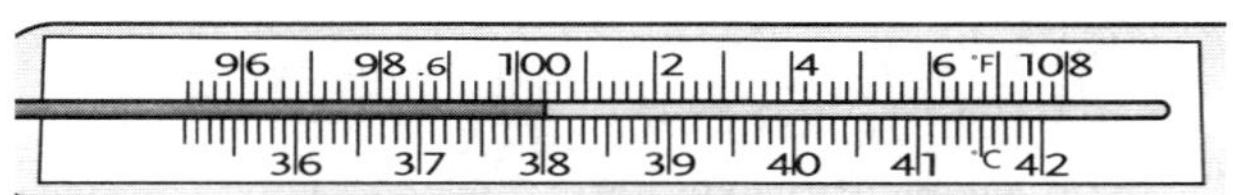

11. ______________________________

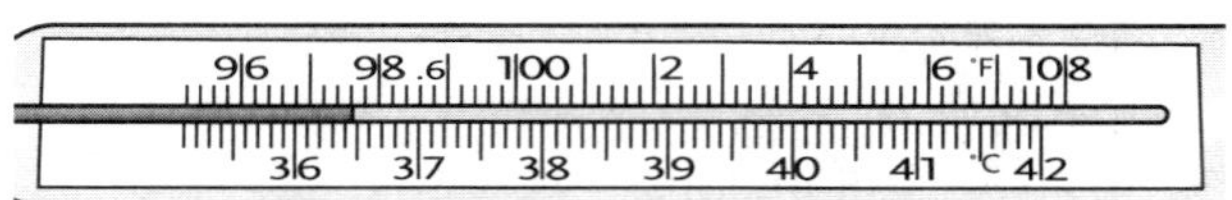

12. ______________________________

Multiple Choice

13. A rectal thermometer is usually color-coded
    (A) Green
    (B) Red
    (C) Black
    (D) Blue

14. Which of the following is the normal temperature range for the oral method?
    (A) 90.6–94.6 degrees Fahrenheit
    (B) 93.6–97.9 degrees Fahrenheit
    (C) 97.6–99.6 degrees Fahrenheit
    (D) 98.6–100.6 degrees Fahrenheit

15. Which of the following temperature sites is another word for the armpit area?
    (A) Temporal artery
    (B) Rectum
    (C) Axilla
    (D) Tympanum

16. Which temperature site is considered to be the most accurate?
    (A) Mouth
    (B) Rectum
    (C) Temporal artery
    (D) Ear

17. How long do digital thermometers take to display a person's temperature?
    (A) 2 to 60 seconds
    (B) 1 to 2 minutes
    (C) 3 minutes
    (D) Less than 1 second

18. How are temporal artery thermometers used to measure body temperature?
    (A) The thermometer is inserted into the person's mouth and under the tongue for approximately 1 minute.
    (B) The thermometer is scanned across the forehead.
    (C) The thermometer is placed in the axillary area for 8 to 10 minutes.
    (D) The thermometer is inserted ¼ inch into the ear.

Fill in the Blank

19. To convert temperatures from Celsius to Fahrenheit, (°C x _____) + _____ = °F.

20. To convert temperatures from Fahrenheit to Celsius, (°F – _____) ÷ _____ = °C.

21. A parent reports that his child's fever was 103°F during the night. How would the MA document this temperature in Celsius?

    _____

22. During intake, a patient sees that her temperature measures 38°C. She asks what that is in Fahrenheit. What is the correct answer?

    _____

Matching

Match each term to the correct definition below. Use each letter only once.

23. _____ Cyanosis

24. _____ Diaphoresis

25. _____ Pallor

26. _____ Turgor

(A) A gray or bluish tint to the skin

(B) Elasticity of the skin

(C) Extreme sweating

(D) Skin tone that is lighter than normal for the patient

7. List guidelines for measuring pulse, respirations, and oxygen saturation

Multiple Choice

1. Where is the apical pulse located?
   (A) Just below the ankle
   (B) On the inside of the wrist
   (C) On the inside of the elbow
   (D) On the left side of the chest, just below the nipple

2. What is the most common site for monitoring the pulse rate?
   (A) Apical pulse
   (B) Femoral pulse
   (C) Pedal pulse
   (D) Radial pulse

3. The medical term for difficulty breathing is
   (A) Dyspeptic
   (B) Dysphagia
   (C) Dyspnea
   (D) Dystolic

4. Which of the following is an instrument that can listen to sounds within the body?
   (A) Reflex hammer
   (B) Scalpel
   (C) Stethoscope
   (D) Microscope

Name: ____________________

5. Inhaling air into the lungs is called
   (A) Inspiration
   (B) Expiration
   (C) Rhythm
   (D) Pulse

6. Exhaling air out of the lungs is called
   (A) Inspiration
   (B) Expiration
   (C) Rhythm
   (D) Pulse

7. The normal respiration rate for adults ranges from
   (A) 5 to 10 breaths per minute
   (B) 12 to 20 breaths per minute
   (C) 25 to 32 breaths per minute
   (D) 7 to 11 breaths per minute

8. Why is it important for the MA to observe respirations without letting the patient know what she is doing?
   (A) People may breathe more quickly if they know they are being observed.
   (B) People will hold their breath if they know what an MA wants to measure.
   (C) The procedure takes less time if the patient is unaware of what is happening.
   (D) Observing respirations is a painful process for most people.

9. What words may be used to describe pulse volume?
   (A) Minimal, sufficient, or excessive
   (B) Adequate, excellent, or uncontrolled
   (C) Thin, robust, or extreme
   (D) Weak, strong, or bounding

10. What is the easiest site to use when measuring pulse in infants and small children?
    (A) Apical pulse
    (B) Femoral pulse
    (C) Pedal pulse
    (D) Radial pulse

11. Another term for blood oxygen level is
    (A) Pulse-ox
    (B) Oxygen saturation
    (C) Suffusion
    (D) RBC sat

12. What may have to be removed to get an accurate reading on a pulse oximeter?
    (A) Rings on the finger being used
    (B) Long-sleeved shirts or blouses
    (C) Nail polish on the finger being used
    (D) All metal jewelry

8. Explain guidelines for measuring blood pressure

Short Answer

For each of the gauges shown below, record the blood pressure shown and answer the question.

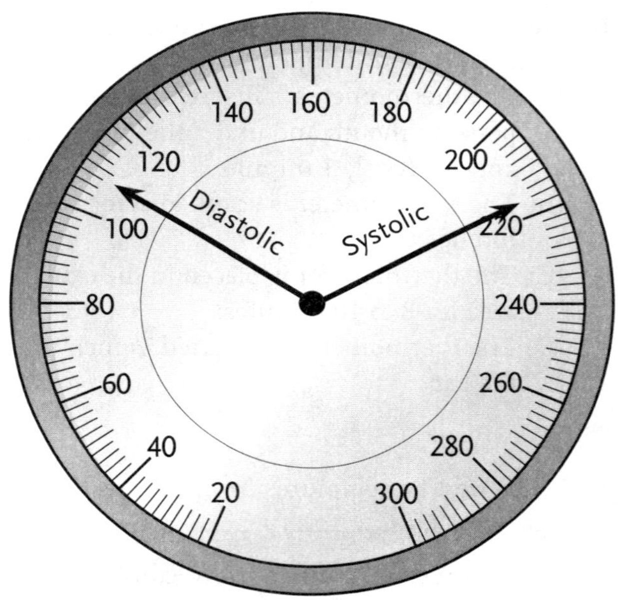

1. ____________________

   Is this reading within normal range?

   ____

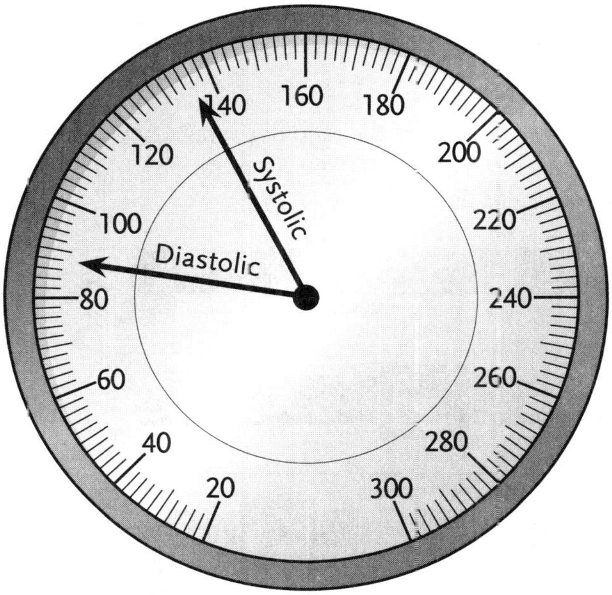

2. ______________________

Is this reading within normal range?

____

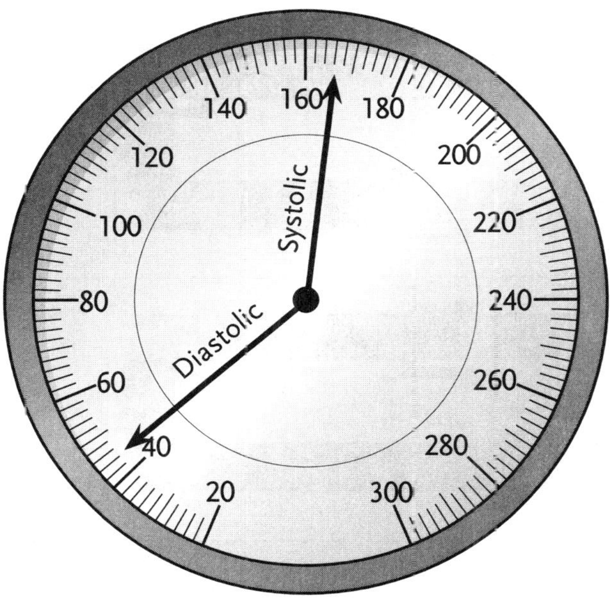

3. ______________________

Is this reading within normal range?

____

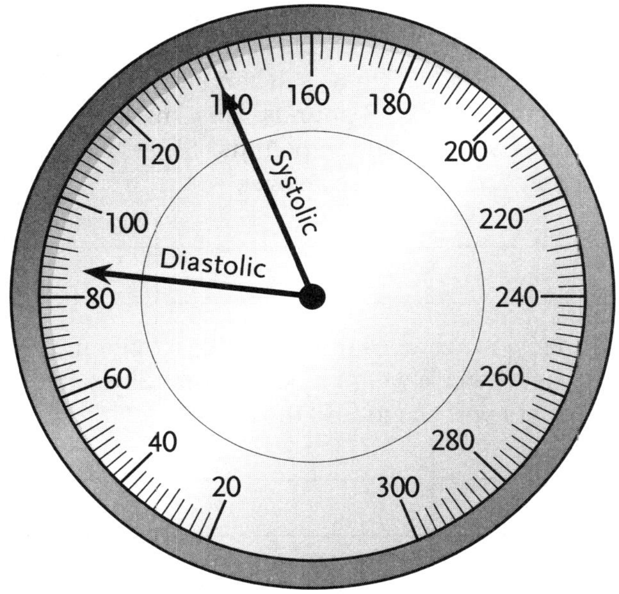

4. ______________________

Is this reading within normal range?

____

9. Describe guidelines for measuring height, weight, and infant head circumference

Short Answer

1. How often is height measured for a pediatric patient?

____

2. How often is weight measured? Why should any gain or loss be reported?

____

____

____

____

3. What must an MA do at all times while weighing an infant?

____

____

Name: ______________________________

4. A patient who uses a wheelchair is rolled onto a wheelchair scale and the reading is 203 pounds. The wheelchair's label indicates that it weighs 43 pounds. How much does the patient weigh in pounds? Show the math you use to find the answer.

____

____

5. How much does the person described in the last exercise weigh in kilograms? Show the math you use to find the answer.

____

____

6. How many centimeters are in one meter?

____

7. If a patient's height measures 190 centimeters, how tall is that person in feet and inches? Show the math you use to find the answer.

____

____

8. If a patient's height measures 5 feet, 7 inches, how tall is that person in meters? Show the math you use to find the answer.

____

____

Fill in the Blank

9. Since infants are unable to stand, infant height is generally referred to as ____________.

10. Growth charts are used to document infant growth from ____________ to ____________.

11. The MA measures an infant's ____________ circumference at each visit. The measurement is used to screen for ____________.

12. BMI is calculated by dividing a person's ____________ in kilograms by the square of their ____________ in meters.

13. Increased weight in the ____________ of the body has been associated with heart disease.

Labeling

Looking at each of the readings shown below, determine each patient's weight for questions 14 to 17 and height for questions 18 to 21.

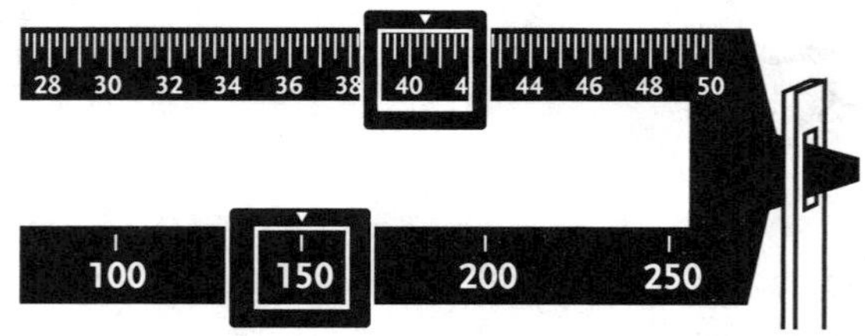

14. ______________________________

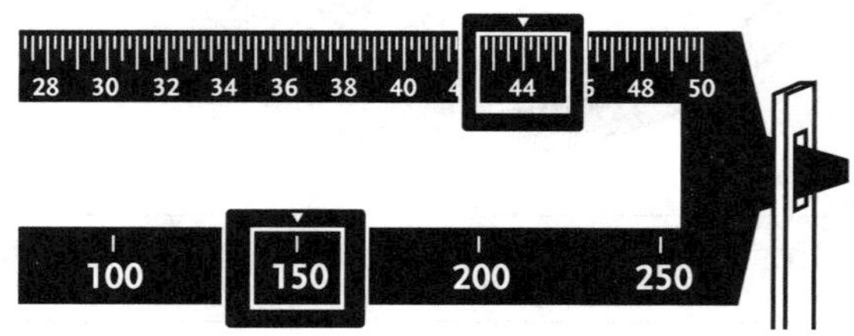

15. ______________________________

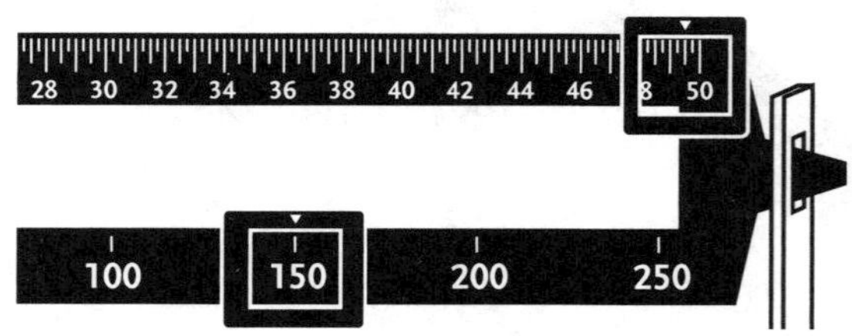

16. ______________________________

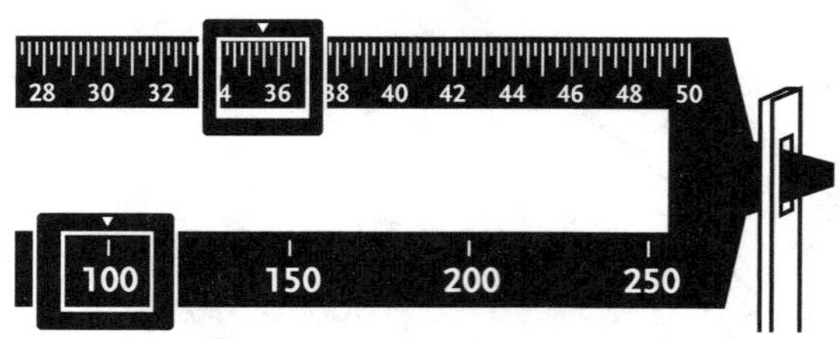

17. ______________________________

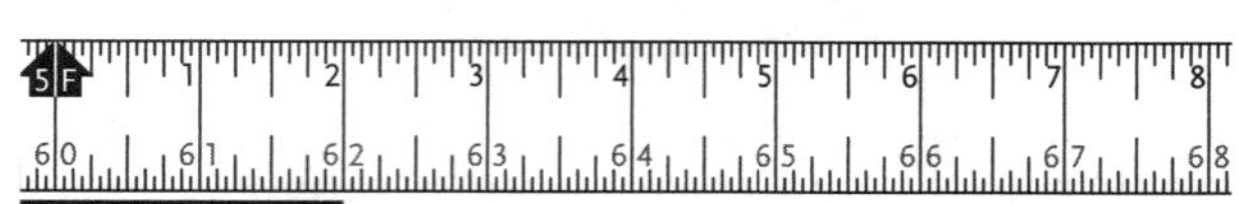

18. ______________________________

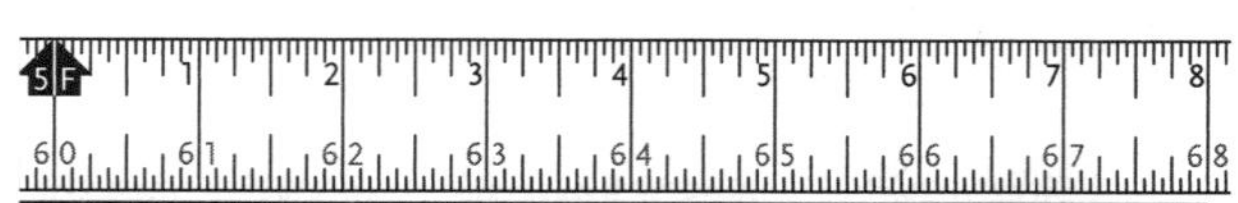

19. ______________________________

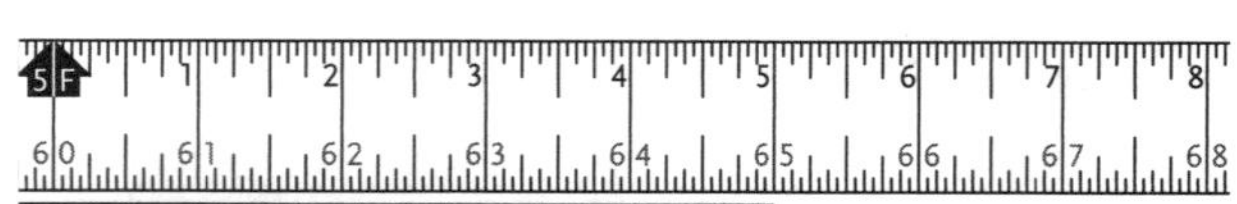

20. ______________________________

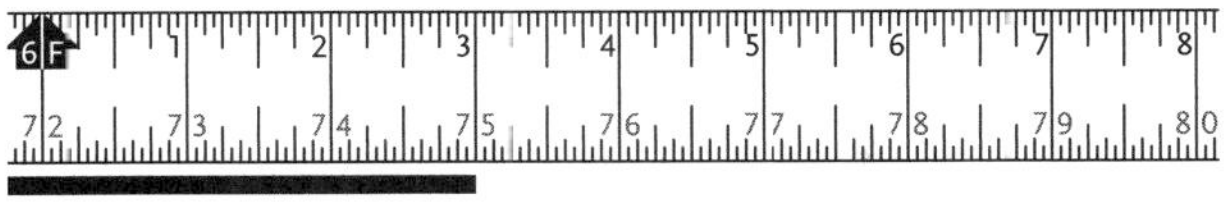

21. ______________________________

10. Explain methods for measuring and reporting pain levels

True or False

1. ____ It is normal for pain to increase with age.
2. ____ An MA should decide how much pain a patient is experiencing and use the MA's words to describe it in the patient's records.
3. ____ Pain that is not relieved in some way can lead to withdrawal, depression, and isolation.
4. ____ Pain can be measured objectively, like blood pressure or body temperature.
5. ____ A patient's pain levels should be checked at every encounter.

Short Answer

6. For each letter of the mnemonic *PQRST*, list the word(s) it represents and list one question related to it.

____

____

____

____

____

____

____

____

____

____

7. List five reasons a patient may not want to report pain.

____

____

____

____

____

____

____

____

8. List six things an MA should report that may relate to patient pain.

____

____

____

____

____

____

____

11. Describe how to position and drape patients for examination

Matching

Match descriptions to the correct position. Letters may be used more than once.

1. ____ The patient lies on their abdomen.
2. ____ This position may be used to examine patients who have shortness of breath when lying flat.
3. ____ This position is often used to examine the thorax, abdomen, and perineum.
4. ____ The patient is face-down with the buttocks raised and their chest and knees supporting their body.

5. ____ The patient is reclining with the head elevated between 45 and 60 degrees.
6. ____ This position is used for a gynecological examination.
7. ____ The patient lies on the left side with the right knee raised toward the chest.
8. ____ The patient lies flat on their back.
9. ____ The patient lies flat on their back with their knees flexed and feet flat on the exam table.
10. ____ This position may be used for a routine physical examination.
11. ____ The patient lies face-up with the legs spread and supported in stirrups.

(A) Seated
(B) Fowler's
(C) Supine
(D) Dorsal recumbent
(E) Prone
(F) Lithotomy
(G) Lateral
(H) Sims'
(I) Knee-chest

12. Describe preparations for surgical procedures in an outpatient setting

Short Answer

1. List four procedures commonly performed in an outpatient medical clinic.

______
______
______
______
______

2. What are the steps needed to prepare a procedure room to the level of surgical asepsis?

______
______
______
______
______

3. What does it mean to prepare a sterile field?

______
______
______
______
______

4. List five items that may be found on a biopsy tray.

______
______
______
______
______

Fill in the Blank

5. When cleaning an exam room surface with bleach, the MA should use a(n) ______ mixture of bleach and water.
6. Contaminated instruments should be completely covered in bactericidal solution for ______ minutes.
7. Scissors and other hinged instruments should be placed in a(n) ______ position to dry.
8. When performing sterile wrapping, the wrap should be placed on a(n) ______ surface in the shape of a(n) ______.

9. After wrapping instruments for sterilization, the MA should write ________________ and their ________________ on the tape with permanent marker.

10. A dry heat autoclave may be used for instruments that may ________________ when exposed to steam.

11. When using an autoclave, bowls and cups should be placed on ________________.

12. Packages are considered sterile for ________________ after autoclaving.

True or False

13. ____ Jewelry can be left on during a surgical scrub if it is flat and smooth, without any grooves or designs.

14. ____ A surgical scrub always moves away from the fingertips.

15. ____ A scrub brush is used to produce a lather during a surgical scrub.

16. ____ After scrubbing is complete, the rinse for a surgical scrub should be done with fingers pointing downward.

17. ____ After a surgical scrub, the hands should be held naturally at the sides of the body.

18. ____ All surfaces of sterile gloves are considered to be sterile.

19. ____ The dominant hand is inserted into the first sterile glove.

20. ____ The first step to putting on the second sterile glove is to insert the fingers of the gloved hand under the folded cuff of the second glove.

21. ____ The outer 3 inches around a sterile field are considered nonsterile.

22. ____ The drop method is used to add all items to the sterile field.

Multiple Choice

23. What should an MA do before adding any liquid to a sterilized bowl?
    (A) Smell the liquid to make sure it is not spoiled
    (B) Shake the liquid to make sure it is properly mixed
    (C) Read the SDS for the liquid to understand what chemicals it contains
    (D) Pour some of the liquid into a sink or other container to decontaminate the rim of the bottle

24. When arranging sterile items on a sterile field, where should sharp instruments such as scalpels be placed?
    (A) In the outer 2 inches of the field
    (B) Underneath a small sterile towel
    (C) In an easily visible location
    (D) At the closest edge of the field

25. Which of the following is something that could be placed on the sterile field using the drop method?
    (A) A gauze pad
    (B) A bowl filled with antiseptic
    (C) A scalpel
    (D) A pair of scissors

26. Where should bowls for solutions be placed on a sterile field?
    (A) In the center
    (B) On top of lightweight items such as gauze to ensure the lightweight items are not blown off
    (C) On the edge
    (D) Right next to any sharp instruments

27. What is important for an MA to know regarding surgical procedures?
    (A) How to prepare for procedures common at their facility and the preferences of the provider they work for
    (B) How to prepare for all types of surgical procedures that may be performed at any facility
    (C) How to perform each step of common surgical procedures
    (D) The name and cause of all conditions that may require a surgical procedure

13. Describe the medical assistant's role during outpatient surgical procedures

Fill in the Blank

1. Patient identification must use at least ______________________ identifiers.
2. If an armband is not used, a(n) ______________________ or ______________________ can verify identity.
3. A(n) ______________________ consent document must be signed before any procedure begins.
4. Preoperative instructions may include ______________, or having nothing by mouth (________) before the procedure, cleaning the __________________ with an antiseptic, or stopping some ____________ prior to the surgery.
5. Before a surgical procedure, the MA should review __________________ and medications with the patient.
6. He should ask if the patient would like to use ______________________.
7. The MA should provide a(n) ______________ and ________________ if clothing needs to be removed.
8. The patient's position during surgery is determined by ______________________.
9. A surgical site is cleaned in a(n) ______________________ process using ____________ different cleaning agents.
10. After a surgical site is cleaned, it should be allowed to ______________ before draping.

Matching

Match each phrase to one of the surgical tools/items. Letters may be used more than once.

11. ____ Used to pull back the edges of a surgical incision
12. ____ Used to clamp blood vessels
13. ____ Disposable ones must be discarded in a sharps container.
14. ____ May be used to handle dressings or grasp body tissues
15. ____ Creates a surgical incision
16. ____ Closes a surgical incision
17. ____ Some have a scissor-like appearance and lock in place; others have a single side and are held in place by hand.
18. ____ Staples may be used instead of these.

(A) Scalpel

(B) Hemostats

(C) Forceps

(D) Retractors

(E) Sutures

Short Answer

19. In what direction should a surgical wound be cleaned before applying a sterile dressing?

____

____

20. After cleaning a surgical wound, what should the MA do before applying sterile gauze pads?

____

____

21. After applying a sterile dressing, what should the MA document?

____

____

____

22. List five things that may be included in postoperative instructions for a patient.

____

____

____

____

____

____

____

23. When are sutures or staples removed?

____

____

14. Understand how tests and diagnostic procedures are ordered and how results are reported

Multiple Choice

1. What may be given to a patient to submit when he goes for a diagnostic test?
   (A) A computer disk with details about the test
   (B) A paper requisition detailing the ordered test
   (C) The provider's business card
   (D) A link to an electronic requisition

2. What must an MA do with test results received in paper form if the office uses electronic records?
   (A) Call the testing facility and request electronic results
   (B) Scan the results and post them to the proper section of the patient's EHR
   (C) Type the results into the proper section of the patient's EHR and then put the paper in a recycling bin
   (D) Type the results into the proper section of the patient's EHR and then shred the paper

3. What should an MA do if she receives a call saying that a patient's lab results are dangerously out of range?
   (A) Call the patient immediately and provide the results
   (B) Ask to speak with the caller's supervisor to confirm the results
   (C) Call the patient and tell her to return to the lab for a new test to confirm the results
   (D) Immediately direct the call to the provider

4. Which of the following is within an MA's scope of practice?
   (A) Answering a patient's questions about the medical cause of abnormal test results
   (B) Making a diagnosis based on a patient's test results
   (C) Communicating instructions from the provider related to diet or lifestyle changes based on test results
   (D) Answering a patient's questions about different medications the patient may take to improve abnormal test results

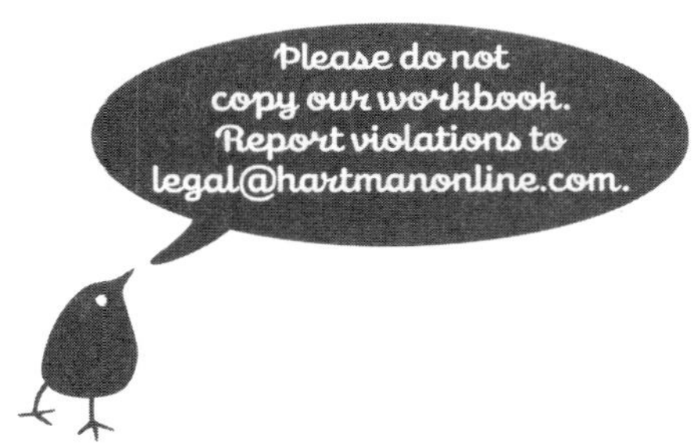

Name: ______________________________

14

The Integumentary System and Related Care

1. Describe the structure and function of the integumentary system

Fill in the Blank

1. The largest organ and system in the body is the ______________________________.
2. Skin prevents ______________________________ to internal organs.
3. Skin also prevents the loss of too much ______________________________.
4. The skin is a(n)________________ organ that feels heat, cold, pain, touch, and pressure.
5. Blood vessels ______________________________, or widen, when the outside temperature is too high.
6. Blood vessels ______________________________, or narrow, when the outside temperature is too cold.

2. Discuss lifespan changes to the integumentary system

Normal or Sign/Symptom

Determine which of the following is a normal lifespan change in an older adult patient and which should be documented in the patient's record as a sign/symptom. Write N for normal aging or S for a sign/symptom.

1. ____ Thinning skin
2. ____ Bruises
3. ____ Wounds
4. ____ Wrinkles
5. ____ Brown spots
6. ____ Thinning of fatty tissue
7. ____ Rashes or flaking of skin
8. ____ Thinning hair
9. ____ Less elastic skin
10. ____ Color changes in skin
11. ____ Swelling
12. ____ Drier skin
13. ____ Redness or discoloration between the toes

3. List common chronic and acute conditions of the integumentary system

Labeling

Label the skin lesions in the illustration using letters from the list that follows.

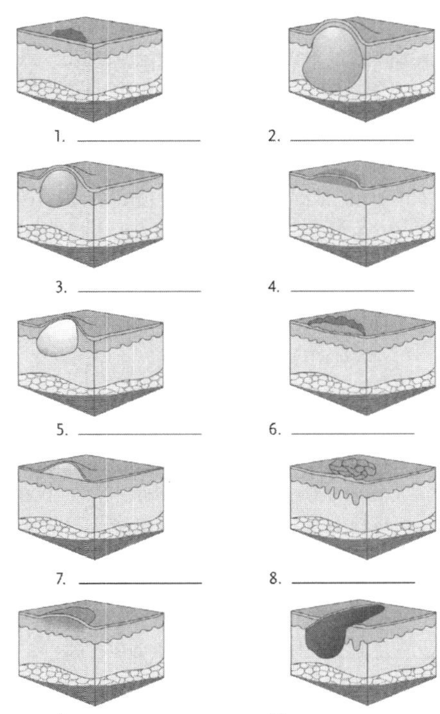

Name: ______________________________

(A) Crust
(B) Wheal
(C) Macule
(D) Ulcer
(E) Pustule
(F) Papule
(G) Scale
(H) Nodule
(I) Vesicle
(J) Plaque

Matching

Use each letter only once.

11. ____ Dermatitis
12. ____ Fungal infection
13. ____ Scabies
14. ____ Shingles
15. ____ Wound

(A) Caused by fungal imbalances; athlete's foot, vaginal yeast infections, and ringworm are examples

(B) Contagious skin infection caused by a mite that burrows into the skin, where it lays eggs, causing intense itching and a skin rash

(C) A type of injury to the skin; classified as either closed or open

(D) Skin rash caused by the varicella-zoster virus (VZV), which is the same virus that causes chickenpox

(E) A general term that refers to an inflammation, or swelling, of the skin

Fill in the Blank

16. A(n) ______________________ has a rapid onset; this type of illness is usually short-term and is treated immediately. A(n) ______________________ is long-term or long-lasting, even lasting over a lifetime.

17. The ______________ of a disease is its origin or cause.

18. ______________ are doctors who specialize in conditions of the integumentary system.

19. ______________ is an infestation of lice. It is very important to locate and remove ______________ (lice eggs) from the hair.

20. __________ is a four-letter acronym for a type of staphylococcus that can cause cellulitis. It is especially __________ to treat.

21. There are three types of skin cancer: __________ cell carcinoma, __________ cell carcinoma, and malignant __________.

22. BCC appears as a new flat or ______________ growth that may be sore or red. It may ______________.

23. SCC is less common than BCC but is more likely to ______________.

24. ____________________________ is the most dangerous type of skin cancer. Lesions are ________________ (one side does not mirror the other) and have ______________ borders.

Short Answer

25. What type of bacteria can infect wounds and make them very difficult to heal? How can MAs help prevent this from happening?

____

____

____

____

____

26. How might rosacea appear in patients with dark skin tones?

____

____

____

____

____

____

27. List a condition of the integumentary system that is also an autoimmune condition. How is this condition treated?

____

____

____

____

____

____

28. What causes stasis dermatitis? List three signs/symptoms of this condition.

____

____

____

____

____

4. Describe examinations and procedures related to the integumentary system

Multiple Choice

1. What type of light does a Wood's light use to detect skin abnormalities?
   (A) X-ray
   (B) Ultraviolet
   (C) Infrared
   (D) Gamma

2. What is the name of the instrument with a circular lens that magnifies skin lesions for closer inspection?
   (A) Dermatoscope
   (B) Wood's light
   (C) Magnifying glass
   (D) Microscope

3. The provider may ask an MA to do these things if skin lesions are found:
   (A) Excise and bandage
   (B) Abrade and dress
   (C) Assess and diagnose
   (D) Photograph and measure

4. Who determines when staples or sutures are ready to be removed?
   (A) The MA
   (B) The patient
   (C) A nurse
   (D) The provider

5. How far should a suture knot be lifted before the suture is snipped?
   (A) Just enough to slip the scissors under the suture
   (B) Until the pressure causes the suture to break
   (C) Approximately 1 centimeter
   (D) Approximately 1 inch

6. Which of the following is an example of aesthetic dermatology?
   (A) Removal of a mole
   (B) Biopsy of a suspicious skin lesion
   (C) Suturing of a laceration
   (D) Botox injections

5. Discuss patient education related to the integumentary system

Short Answer

1. A patient has recently moved to a new area with a much drier climate than she is used to. She is worried about her skin, which has been dry, itchy, and easily irritated. A dermatologist examines the patient and does not find any sign of illness or injury. She asks her MA to send the patient a message in the patient portal listing ways to prevent drying and irritation. What are three suggestions the MA could list?

____

____

____

____

____

____

____

Name: ______________________________

2. If an MA is assigned to provide patient education about sun exposure and use of sunscreen, what are two of the most important points to include?

3. List three nutrients that are related to skin health and describe the benefit they provide.

4. When should a patient seek medical care for a puncture wound?

5. What do the letters *ABCDE* stand for in relation to skin observation?

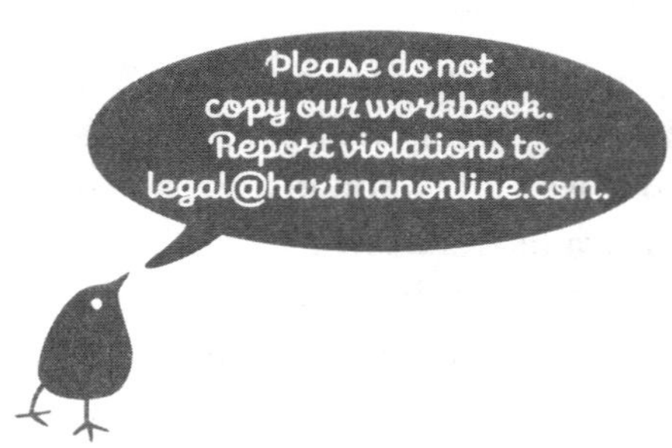

Name: ______________________________

15

The Musculoskeletal System and Related Care

1. Describe the structure and function of the musculoskeletal system

True or False

1. ____ The body is shaped by muscles, bones, ligaments, tendons, and cartilage.
2. ____ The human body has 215 bones.
3. ____ Bones are made up of dead cells.
4. ____ Bones protect the body's organs.
5. ____ Hematopoiesis, or the production of red blood cells, happens in the muscles.
6. ____ Two bones meet at a joint.
7. ____ A hinge joint, such as the elbow, can bend in two directions.
8. ____ Cartilaginous joints do not allow any movement.
9. ____ Muscles allow movement of body parts.
10. ____ Skeletal muscles are involuntary muscles.
11. ____ The heart is an involuntary muscle.
12. ____ Skeletal muscles are covered by a tough, sheet-like connective tissue called an agonist.

Labeling

For each of the following illustrations, write the correct term for the body movement shown.

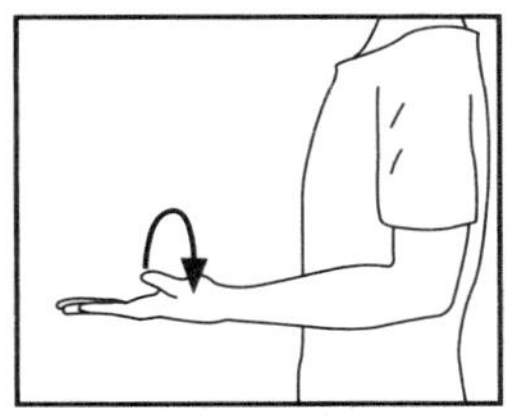

13. ______________________

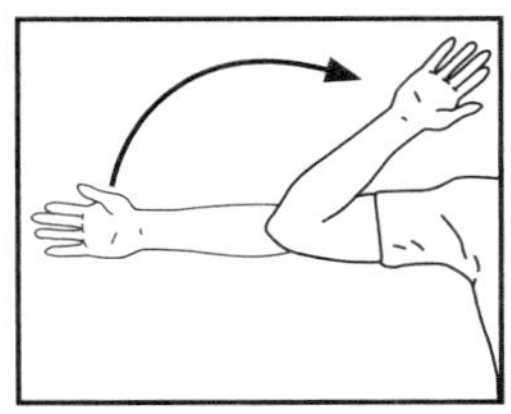

14. ______________________

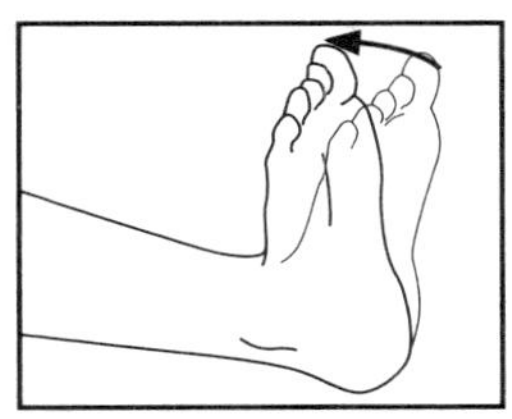

15. ______________________

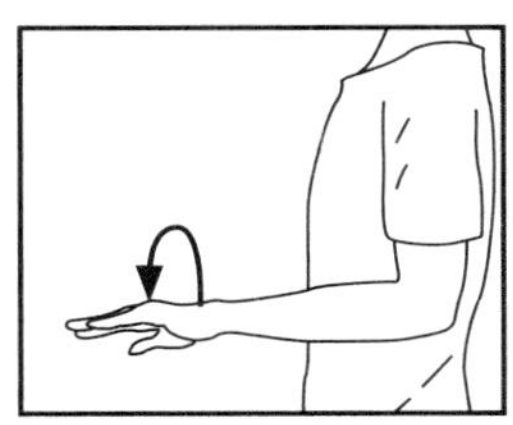

16. ______________________

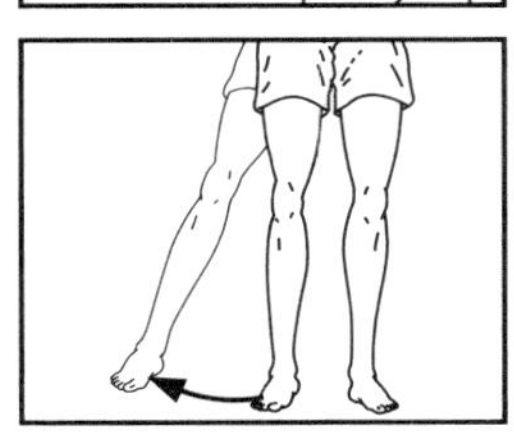

17. ______________________

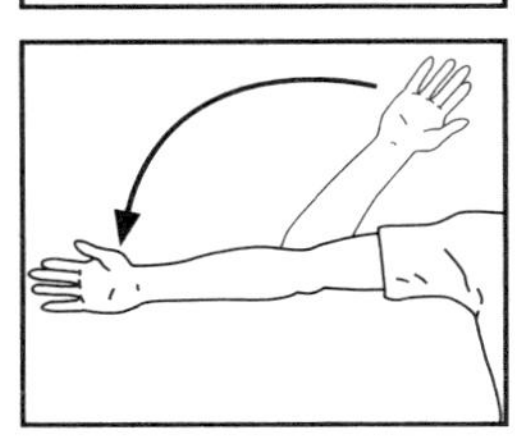

18. ______________________

Name: ________________________________

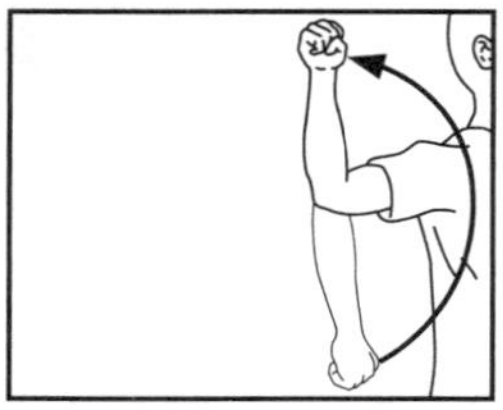

19. ____________________

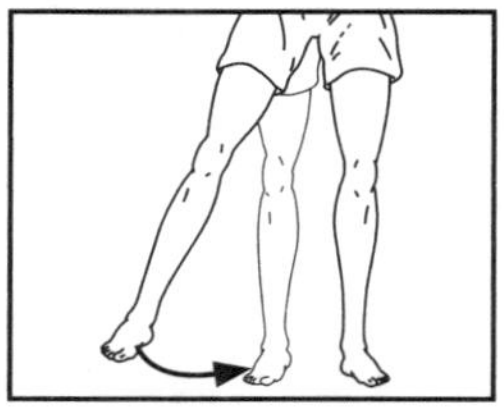

20. ____________________

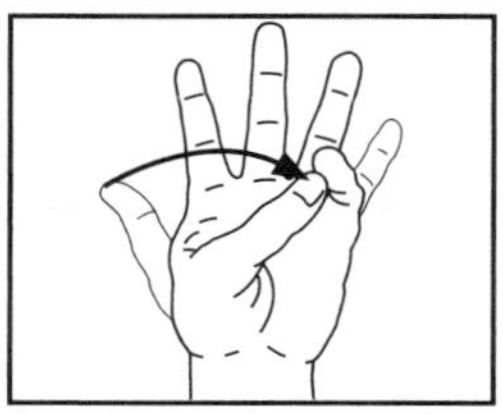

21. ____________________

2. Discuss lifespan changes to the musculoskeletal system

Normal or Sign/Symptom

Determine which of the following is normal and which should be documented in the patient's record as a sign/symptom. Assume the patient is an adult over 50 unless otherwise stated. Write N *for normal or* S *for a sign/symptom.*

1. _____ Bruising
2. _____ Slow weakening of muscles
3. _____ Some soft bones in a newborn infant
4. _____ Gradual loss of muscle tone
5. _____ Stiff joints after inactivity
6. _____ Sharp pain during movement
7. _____ Inability to tie shoelaces in a 1-year-old child
8. _____ Increased swelling of joints
9. _____ White, shiny, warm, or red/discolored areas over a joint
10. _____ Inability to sit up in a 1-year-old child

3. List common chronic and acute conditions of the musculoskeletal system

Inflammatory/Bone-Deteriorating Disorders

Multiple Choice

1. Arthritis is a general term referring to ______ of the joints.
   (A) Immobility
   (B) Inflammation
   (C) Redness
   (D) Stiffness

2. Arthritis may be the result of
   (A) Congestive heart failure
   (B) Amputation
   (C) Autoimmune illness
   (D) Substance abuse

3. Osteoarthritis is common in
   (A) The elderly
   (B) Infants
   (C) Teenagers
   (D) Adults in their 20s and 30s

4. Pain and stiffness of osteoarthritis may increase with
   (A) Hot weather
   (B) Cold weather
   (C) An active lifestyle
   (D) Intake of fluids

5. Rheumatoid arthritis affects the _______ joints first.
   (A) Smaller
   (B) Larger
   (C) Elbow
   (D) There is no typical progression.

6. The type of doctor who usually treats rheumatoid arthritis is a(n)
   (A) Orthopedic specialist
   (B) Rheumatologist
   (C) Podiatrist
   (D) Gerontologist

7. Arthritis is generally treated with
   (A) Surgical removal of the affected limb
   (B) Application of a cast to immobilize the affected area
   (C) Deep breathing exercises
   (D) Anti-inflammatory medications

Name: ______________________________

8. This condition is caused by the painful buildup of uric acid crystals in the joints:
   (A) Rheumatoid arthritis
   (B) Gout
   (C) Osteomalacia
   (D) Lordosis

9. A DEXA scan is used to diagnose
   (A) Osteoarthritis
   (B) Plantar fasciitis
   (C) Scoliosis
   (D) Osteoporosis

10. Osteomalacia is usually caused by a severe deficiency of
   (A) Vitamin D
   (B) Vitamin C
   (C) Calcium
   (D) Iron

Curvature Disorders

Labeling

Label the curvature disorders in the illustration using letters from the list that follows.

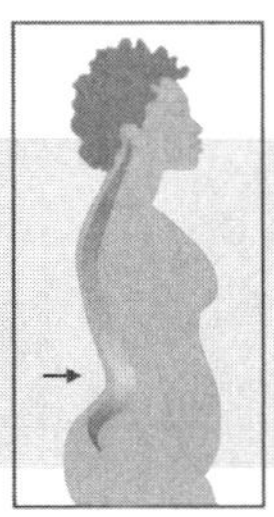

11. ____________

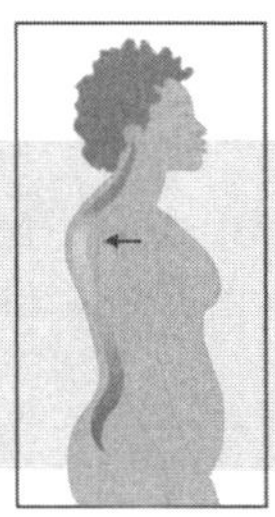

12. ____________

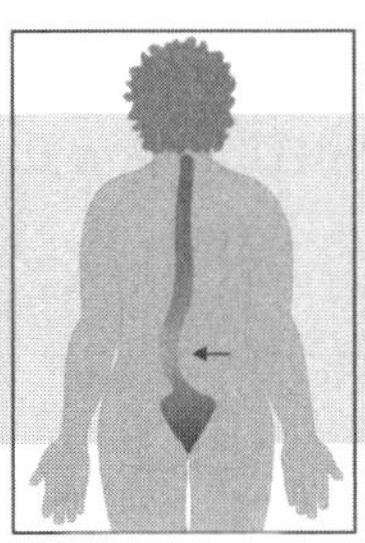

13. ____________

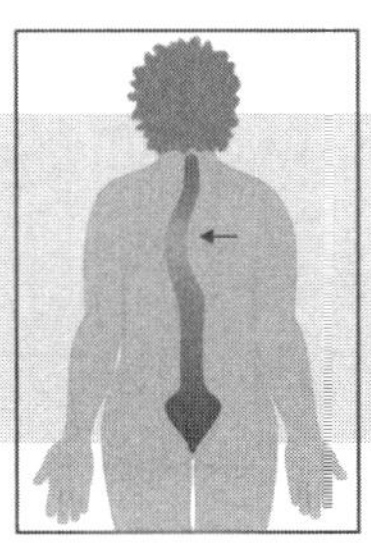

14. ____________

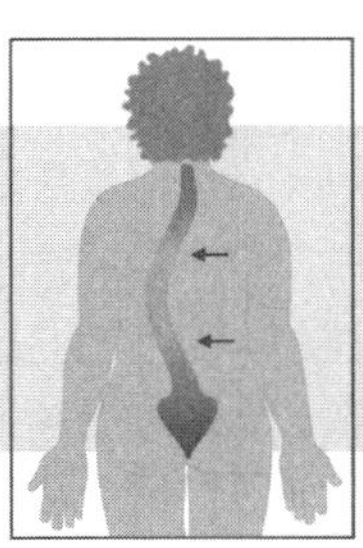

15. ____________

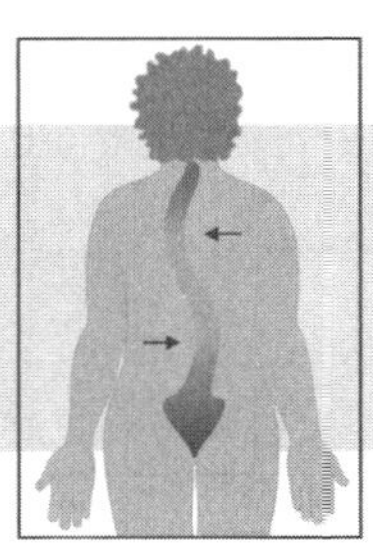

16. ____________

(A) Thoracolumbar scoliosis

(B) Thoracic scoliosis

(C) Lordosis

(D) Lumbar scoliosis

(E) Combined scoliosis

(F) Kyphosis

Injury-Related Disorders

Fill in the Blank

17. When a vertebra is injured it may put pressure on the intervertebral disc and cause it to bulge, or ________________.

18. Back pain is a leading cause of ________________________.

19. Activity-related stress results from standing or sitting for long periods of time, improper body ______________, or poor ____________ mechanics.

20. Treatment of back pain depends on the ___________. It may include rest, analgesics, ___________ exercises, and physical therapy.

21. Muscle ______________ are caused by an injury to a muscle or tendon. Joint ______________ are caused by injury to a joint or ligament.

Matching

Match each term to a definition below. Use each letter only once.

22. ____ Closed fracture

23. ____ Open (compound) fracture

24. ____ Displaced fracture

25. ____ Nondisplaced fracture

26. ____ Greenstick fracture

27. ____ Transverse fracture

28. ____ Linear (longitudinal) fracture

29. ____ Oblique fracture

30. ____ Spiral fracture

31. ____ Comminuted fracture

32. ____ Stress (hairline) fracture

33. ____ Compression fracture

34. ____ Depressed fracture

35. ____ Impacted fracture

36. ____ Pathologic fracture

37. ____ Colles fracture

(A) A skull fracture that pushes a segment of cranial bone into the brain beneath

(B) A broken bone that penetrates the skin

(C) A fracture that occurs when the bone is twisted forcefully

(D) A fracture that is due to an underlying disease, such as osteoporosis, weakening the bones

(E) A fracture splintered into many pieces

(F) A fracture in which the bone is broken vertically along the bone's length

(G) A wrist fracture affecting the distal radius

(H) A fracture in which the bone has not moved out of alignment

(I) A broken bone that does not break the skin

(J) A fracture that is pressed downward or smashed; impacts the vertebrae and is common in adults with osteoporosis

(K) A fracture in which bone fragments are pushed inward and pressed into each other

(L) A fracture broken across the horizontal plane, or straight across the bone

(M) A break that has moved out of alignment

(N) A partial fracture common in young children

(O) A slanted break that curves along the bone

(P) A small crack in the bone

Chronic Musculoskeletal Disorders

Short Answer

38. What are some of the body systems, in addition to the musculoskeletal system, affected by fibromyalgia?

____

____

____

39. List four symptoms of fibromyalgia.

____

____

____

____

40. What muscles are most affected by myasthenia gravis?

____

____

____

41. Muscular dystrophy (MD) is a progressive disease. What does that mean?

____

____

____

42. What is the main effect that MD has on the muscles?

____

____

____

43. What does *ALS* stand for and what other name is often used for this disease?

____

____

____

44. How long does the average person live with ALS?

____

____

____

Bone and Muscle Tumors/Amputation

True or False

45. ____ Most bone and muscle tumors are cancerous.

46. ____ Cancerous tumors of the bone, muscle, and cartilage occur most often in children and young adults.

47. ____ Amputation is the surgical removal of a body part.

48. ____ Phantom sensation is a tingling feeling in a limb that is going to be amputated.

49. ____ Phantom limb pain is just in the patient's imagination.

50. ____ A prosthesis is a device constructed to replace a missing body part, such as an eye, arm, or leg.

4. Describe examinations and procedures related to the musculoskeletal system

Multiple Choice

1. MAs who work with patients with musculoskeletal disorders must be trained in
   (A) Diagnosing these disorders
   (B) Assessing the need for physical therapy
   (C) Safely assisting with transfers and ambulation
   (D) Taking X-rays

2. What does a goniometer do?
   (A) Measures the range of motion in a joint
   (B) Measures muscle strength
   (C) Measures bone density
   (D) Measures the speed of muscle reaction

3. What should an MA do if a patient starts to fall?
   (A) Widen his stance, bend his knees, and support the patient as he lowers the patient to the floor
   (B) Widen his stance and position himself to block the patient's fall and keep the patient upright
   (C) Step back so that the patient can fall to the ground without hitting the MA
   (D) Step closer and place his arms around the patient to stop the fall

4. Hemiparesis and hemiplegia affect
   (A) One side of the body, left or right
   (B) One half of the body, top or bottom
   (C) One limb
   (D) One body system

5. When is a cane useful?
   (A) When a patient can bear weight on only one leg
   (B) When a patient can bear weight on both legs but needs help with balance
   (C) When a patient has had a limb amputated
   (D) When a patient is fully mobile and has good balance

6. Where should the top of a crutch be in comparison to the patient's axilla?
   (A) 2–3 finger-widths below
   (B) 2–3 finger-widths above
   (C) Fit snugly just below
   (D) A hand-width below

7. When using properly fitted crutches, how should the patient's elbow be positioned?
   (A) Bent at a 90-degree angle
   (B) Bent at a 45-degree angle
   (C) Bent slightly
   (D) Completely straight

8. Thermotherapy and cryotherapy use ____________ and ____________ to treat musculoskeletal injuries.
   (A) Medications, soaks
   (B) Elevation, rest
   (C) Heat, cold
   (D) Rest, gentle motion

9. What is the longest time an MA should use a hot or cold treatment with a patient?
   (A) 10 minutes
   (B) 20 minutes
   (C) 30 minutes
   (D) 1 hour

10. Which of the following exercises are done by the patient with help from a healthcare worker?
   (A) Strength-building
   (B) Active range of motion
   (C) Active assisted range of motion
   (D) Passive range of motion

11. What must be in place before an MA does ROM exercises with a patient?
   (A) An informed consent form
   (B) Sterile asepsis measures
   (C) An order from a provider
   (D) Appropriate athletic shoes

12. What instruments are used during arthrocentesis?
   (A) A reflex hammer and a goniometer
   (B) A scalpel and a small, flexible camera
   (C) Small, needle-like wires and a machine that creates electrical impulses
   (D) A needle and syringe

13. What procedure may be used to aid in the removal of bone fragments or scar tissue from a joint?
   (A) Cryotherapy
   (B) Arthroscopy
   (C) Internal fixation
   (D) Electromyography

Fill in the Blank

14. Casts are applied to ______________ fractures and keep bones in ______________ while they heal.

15. A cast must be completely ______________ before a person can bear weight on it.

16. Before a cast is applied, clean the skin with a(n) __________________________ and allow it to air-dry.

17. Stockinette is applied to a cast site leaving ______________ of extra fabric at each end.

18. ______________ layers of fiberglass roll are applied around a cast.

19. During cast removal, the MA ______________ the patient, ______________ the body part, and ______________ the provider.

20. When applying an elastic bandage, the MA should wrap evenly, from ______________ to ______________.

21. The MA should tell a patient with an elastic bandage to observe for signs of ______________________________, such as numbness, tingling, or skin that is ______________ to the touch.

5. Discuss patient education related to the musculoskeletal system

Matching

Match each item below to the musculoskeletal system benefit described in the textbook. Use each letter only once.

1. ____ Using proper posture and body mechanics
2. ____ Eating carbohydrates
3. ____ Consuming foods or beverages rich in calcium
4. ____ Drinking vitamin D-fortified milk
5. ____ Using gates to restrict access to stairs for babies and toddlers
6. ____ Staying physically active

(A) Maintains the structure and strength of bones

(B) Maintains and improves musculoskeletal health and prevents depression, weakness, and loss of self-esteem

(C) Maintains physical health and prevents injury

(D) Provides energy and maintains muscle strength and endurance

(E) Prevents falls and injuries

(F) Enables the body to absorb calcium

Name: ______________________________

Short Answer

7. What can a patient do to reduce swelling in an extremity with a cast?

____

____

____

8. What should a patient with a cast do if she observes skin discoloration, pressure, and tingling in the extremity with the cast?

____

____

____

9. Why should a patient with a cast not insert anything inside the case (e.g., use a pencil to scratch itchy skin under the cast)?

____

____

____

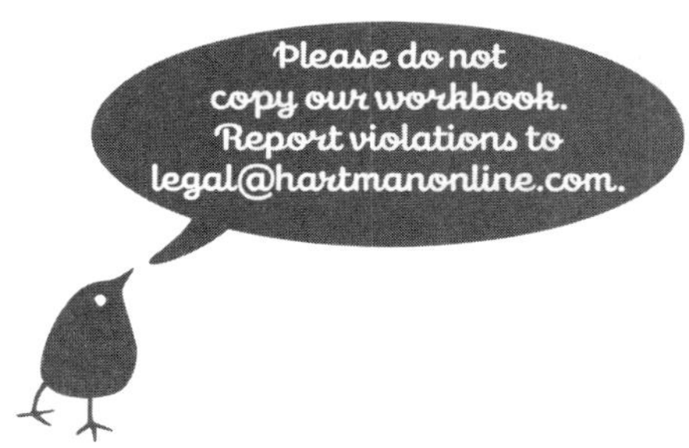

Name: ___________________________

16

The Nervous System and Sense Organs and Related Care

1. Describe the structure and function of the nervous system and sense organs

Multiple Choice

1. The nervous system
   (A) Gives the body shape and structure
   (B) Controls and coordinates body functions
   (C) Is the largest organ in the body
   (D) Pumps blood through the blood vessels to the cells

2. The basic unit of the nervous system is the
   (A) Neuron
   (B) Message
   (C) Brain
   (D) Spinal cord

3. The two main parts of the nervous system are
   (A) The cardiovascular system and integumentary system
   (B) Neurons and receptors
   (C) The body and the brain
   (D) The central nervous system and peripheral nervous system

4. The central nervous system is made up of
   (A) The brain and spinal cord
   (B) Muscles and bones
   (C) Neurons and receptors
   (D) The heart and lungs

5. The peripheral nervous system deals with the outer part of the body via the
   (A) Brain
   (B) Cerebrum
   (C) Nerves
   (D) Right hemisphere

6. What type of chemical carries impulses from neuron to neuron?
   (A) Synapses
   (B) Myelin
   (C) Dendrites
   (D) Neurotransmitters

7. What cushions the brain and spinal cord against injury?
   (A) The nerves
   (B) The spinal column
   (C) The brainstem
   (D) Cerebrospinal fluid

8. The ________ is the part of the brain that controls thinking, speech, and voluntary muscles.
   (A) Brainstem
   (B) Cerebellum
   (C) Cerebral cortex
   (D) Right hemisphere

9. The left hemisphere of the brain controls
   (A) The left side of the body
   (B) The right side of the body
   (C) Both sides of the body
   (D) Memory

10. The brainstem controls
   (A) Smooth movements
   (B) Breathing and swallowing
   (C) Jerky movements
   (D) Emotions and speech

11. The nerve pathways in the spinal cord conduct messages between
   (A) The heart and the blood
   (B) The cerebrum and cerebellum
   (C) The brain and the body
   (D) The muscles and the bones

Short Answer

12. List the five sense organs of the body.

____

____

____

____

____

13. Which part of the eye contains cells that respond to light and send a message to the brain so that a person can see?

____

14. Which nerve communicates these messages from the eye to the brain?

____

15. List the three parts of the ear.

____

____

____

____

2. Discuss lifespan changes to the nervous system and sense organs

Fill in the Blank

1. Newborns are helpless and dependent on others to meet their _______________.
2. Development begins with __________ motor movements, such as rolling over, crawling, and __________.
3. __________ motor movements are mastered next.
4. The very front of the frontal cortex, the ____________ cortex, is the last segment of the brain to mature.
5. Teens may experience _______________ reasoning and __________ impulse control.

Normal or Sign/Symptom

6. ____ Inability to move one side of the body
7. ____ Depression or mood changes
8. ____ Inability to reason in a toddler
9. ____ Fatigue or pain with movement
10. ____ Shaking
11. ____ Decreased sense of taste or smell in a geriatric patient
12. ____ Slurring of speech
13. ____ Impulsive behavior in a teenager
14. ____ Confusion
15. ____ Violent behavior
16. ____ Minor short-term memory loss in a geriatric patient
17. ____ Sudden changes in vision

3. List common chronic and acute conditions of the nervous system and sense organs

Matching

Match each type of provider with the services they provide. Use each letter only once.

1. ____ Neurologist
2. ____ Psychiatrist
3. ____ Clinical psychologist
4. ____ Licensed mental health counselor
5. ____ Licensed social worker
6. ____ Ophthalmologist
7. ____ Optometrist
8. ____ Audiologist
9. ____ Ear, nose, and throat specialist (ENT)

(A) A healthcare provider who diagnoses mental health conditions and treats them with counseling or other therapy

(B) A doctor who manages conditions of the ears and nose as well as disorders of the throat

(C) A physician who diagnoses and treats mental health disorders

(D) A healthcare worker who uses a variety of therapies to treat mental health conditions

(E) A doctor who treats eye diseases and conditions, including performing surgeries

(F) A specialist who treats nervous system disorders, such as stroke or epilepsy

(G) A healthcare worker who provides counseling and support services to patients

(H) A doctor who manages eyesight disorders, such as nearsightedness

(I) A healthcare professional who performs hearing tests and fits patients for hearing aids

Stroke and Nervous System Injuries

True or False

10. _____ A stroke is sometimes called a *brain attack.*

11. _____ A CVA caused by a blockage is called a *hemorrhagic stroke.*

12. _____ Effects from a transient ischemic attack (TIA) usually subside within minutes, but they may last up to 24 hours.

13. _____ A person who has had a TIA is more likely to have a stroke.

14. _____ Physical therapy is not effective for patients who have had strokes.

15. _____ Traumatic brain injury (TBI) is another name for stroke.

16. _____ Effects of a head injury depend on what caused the injury and how severe it is.

17. _____ The higher an injury to the spinal cord, the less loss of function the patient will have.

18. _____ Quadriplegia is a loss of function in the legs, trunk, and arms.

19. _____ A concussion is caused by a banging movement of the brain against the skull.

Degenerative Diseases

Short Answer

20. What is true of an irreversible disease?

____

____

____

21. What is the goal of palliative treatments?

____

____

____

22. What weakens over time for patients with Huntington's disease? What are the goals of treatment?

____

____

____

____

____

____

23. Describe what happens in the brain of a patient with Parkinson's disease. How does this affect the muscles?

____

____

____

____

____

____

24. What happens to the myelin in the nervous system of a patient with multiple sclerosis? How does the disease progress?

____

____

____

25. List five common causes of dementia.

26. What happens in the brain of a patient with Alzheimer's disease to cause dementia?

Pain Disorders/Seizure Disorders

Crossword

Across

28. A journal can help a patient with headaches to identify these.
30. Intensely painful headaches that happen frequently over a period of time, followed by longer stretches of remission
31. A type of headache that can also cause nausea, vomiting, light sensitivity, and visual disturbances
34. Nerve pain caused by irritation, infection, or damage in a nerve
35. A type of headache that causes throbbing pain and may be caused by stress

Down

27. Migraine often has this kind of link.
29. A type of nerve pain also known as *lumbar radiculopathy*
32. A brain disorder that results from a disruption in normal electrical impulses in the brain, causing repeated seizures
33. This kind of seizure happens as a response to a very high body temperature.

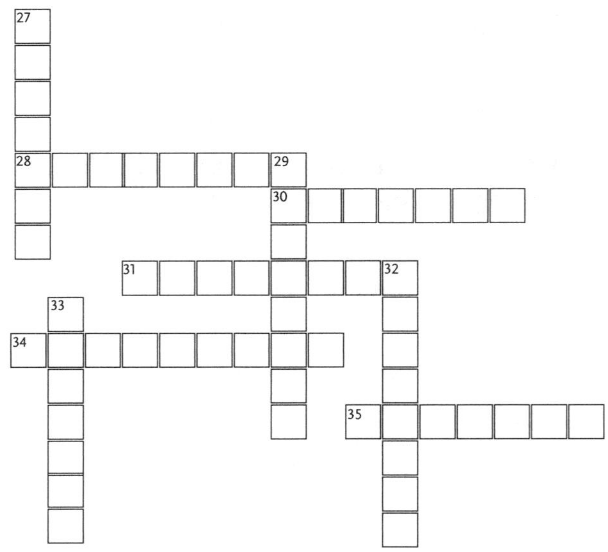

Mental Health Disorders

Fill in the Blank

36. Some conditions caused by physical illness can ______________ mental health disorders.
37. Confusion and ________________, for example, may be related to a mental health disorder but are often symptoms of physical illness.
38. Urinary tract infection (UTI) is a common cause of ______________.
39. Mental health disorders are diagnosed through a(n) ______________________ exam exploring the patient's symptoms, thoughts, and __________________.
40. ______________________________ therapy is a type of psychotherapy in which the therapist helps the patient process their thoughts and feelings so that they can develop their own _____________ mechanisms to manage their symptoms.
41. The provider may also ________________ to treat mental health disorders.

Disorders of the Sense Organs

Matching

Use each letter only once.

42. ____ Presbyopia
43. ____ Cataract
44. ____ Diabetic retinopathy
45. ____ Myopia
46. ____ Age-related macular degeneration
47. ____ Glaucoma
48. ____ Hyperopia
49. ____ Retinal detachment
50. ____ Conjunctivitis
51. ____ Presbycusis
52. ____ Otosclerosis
53. ____ Tinnitus
54. ____ Meniere's disease
55. ____ Perforated eardrum
56. ____ Acute otitis media
57. ____ Cerumen impaction

(A) A ringing or roaring sound in the ears that is not associated with outside sounds

(B) The leading cause of blindness in the US, caused by damaging pressure in the eye

(C) A buildup of earwax

(D) Farsightedness

(E) A condition of the inner ear that causes vertigo, or dizziness and loss of balance

(F) A condition that occurs when part of the retina gradually deteriorates, causing vision loss in the center of the field of vision

(G) A type of hearing impairment that happens gradually with time; caused by hardening of the bones of the middle ear

(H) A form of hyperopia that occurs with aging

(I) A rupture of the tympanic membrane

(J) Nearsightedness

(K) A medical emergency in which the retina pulls away from the back of the eye

(L) A condition in which the lens of the eye becomes cloudy

(M) An infection of the middle ear

(N) A complication of diabetes caused by damage to the retina; can lead to blindness

(O) A form of hearing loss caused by abnormal bone growth in the middle ear

(P) A common and very contagious type of eye infection

4. Describe examinations and procedures related to the nervous system and sense organs

Short Answer

Place a check mark (✓) beside items below that are part of a routine neurological exam.

1. ____ Drawing blood
2. ____ Asking the patient to do jumping jacks
3. ____ Checking mental status by asking questions about their name, where they are, and the date
4. ____ Using tonometry to check pressure in the eyes
5. ____ Using a reflex hammer to test deep tendon reflexes
6. ____ Checking alertness levels by attempting to surprise the patient occasionally during the exam
7. ____ Assessing the patient's ability to balance on a balance beam
8. ____ Using a penlight to check if the patient's pupils constrict when exposed to light and return to normal when it is removed
9. ____ Checking strength by asking the MA to arm-wrestle the patient
10. ____ Measuring sensation by touching the patient

11. ____ Having the patient follow the direction of the provider's finger as she moves it across the patient's visual field

12. ____ Asking the patient to push against the provider's hands to check that the patient's strength is the same on both sides

Multiple Choice

13. MAs may be delegated to use screening tools during intake to help providers identify patients who are experiencing
    (A) Stress or suicidal thoughts
    (B) Seizures
    (C) Stroke symptoms
    (D) Headaches

14. Electromyography measures the ability of muscles to respond to
    (A) Exercise
    (B) Glucose
    (C) Nervous stimuli
    (D) Certain medications

15. Which of the following is a task that may be assigned to an MA during an electroencephalogram (EEG)?
    (A) Placing electrodes on the patient's scalp
    (B) Positioning the patient in the supine position
    (C) Connecting wires to the electrodes
    (D) Making sure the machine is registering the patient's brain activity

16. What may be collected using lumbar puncture?
    (A) A plasma specimen
    (B) A cerumen specimen
    (C) A specimen of fluid from the eye
    (D) A specimen of cerebrospinal fluid

17. The Moro reflex occurs when
    (A) The elbow is hit with a reflex hammer
    (B) An infant curls its fingers around a finger placed on its palm
    (C) An infant turns its head and opens its mouth when its cheek is stroked
    (D) An infant startles and extends its arms outward in response to a sudden position change

Short Answer

18. What are Ishihara plates and what do they test?

____

____

____

____

____

19. What is a Snellen chart used to measure?

____

____

20. What types of charts may be used to screen for myopia in small children or nonreaders?

____

____

____

____

____

21. Describe two types of hearing tests that use tuning forks. Where does the provider place the tuning fork in each test?

____

____

____

____

____

22. What does audiometry measure?

____

____

____

____

____

23. Why might an eye or ear irrigation be performed?

24. Where should the syringe be aimed when irrigating the eye?

25. Where should the syringe be aimed when irrigating the ear?

5. Discuss patient education related to the nervous system and sense organs

Scenarios

1. Tess is a 78-year-old patient who reports that she has been surprised lately by some small slips in her memory. She has also been experiencing stress due to concern about one of her grandchildren, who has been diagnosed with leukemia. MA Stephanie is assigned to provide patient education about keeping the brain stimulated and relieving stress. What may she suggest to Tess?

2. MA Joaquin works at a pediatrician's office. At Cassie's 12-year well check she tells the doctor about all the exciting things she plans to do during her summer vacation: skateboarding, swimming in the pond near her grandma's house, and starting practices with her middle school football team. Joaquin is asked to review injury prevention with Cassie and her mom. What topics should he cover?

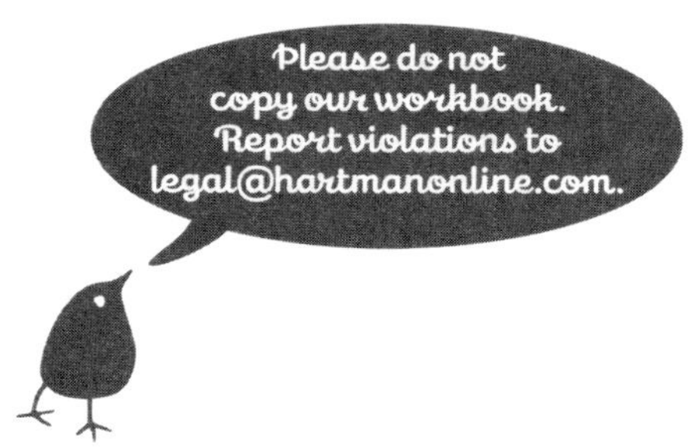

Name: ___________________________________

17

The Circulatory System and Related Care

1. Describe the structure and function of the circulatory system

Multiple Choice

1. What functions as the pump of the circulatory system?
   (A) Heart
   (B) Lungs
   (C) Lymph
   (D) Blood

2. What structure divides the sides of the heart?
   (A) The epicardium
   (B) The aortic valve
   (C) The septum
   (D) The ventricles

3. What are the three layers of the pericardial membrane?
   (A) Inside, middle, and outside
   (B) Proximal, medial, and distal
   (C) Endocardium, myocardium, and epicardium
   (D) Visceral, serous, and fibrous

4. What do the heart's valves do?
   (A) Trigger the pumping action of the heart
   (B) Keep blood flowing in the correct direction
   (C) Move electrical signals through the heart
   (D) Receive nerve impulses

5. Where does the cardiac conduction system begin?
   (A) In the left ventricle
   (B) In the right ventricle
   (C) In the left atrium
   (D) In the right atrium

6. What are the three main types of blood vessels?
   (A) Venules, arterioles, and capillaries
   (B) Arteries, veins, and capillaries
   (C) Visceral, serous, and fibrous
   (D) Oxygenating, deoxygenating, and exchanging

7. Which blood vessels bring oxygenated blood to the heart muscle?
   (A) Pulmonary arteries
   (B) Pulmonary veins
   (C) Coronary arteries
   (D) Superior and inferior venae cavae

8. Which of the following is a type of white blood cell?
   (A) Erythrocyte
   (B) Thrombocyte
   (C) Fibrinogen
   (D) Lymphocyte

9. What is plasma mostly made up of?
   (A) Water
   (B) Oxygen
   (C) Lymph
   (D) Minerals

10. A universal blood donor is a person with the blood type
    (A) O, Rh-negative
    (B) O, Rh-positive
    (C) AB, Rh-positive
    (D) AB, Rh-negative

11. What gives blood its red color?
    (A) Plasma
    (B) Iron
    (C) Lymph
    (D) Glucose

Name: ______________________

12. Which of these terms refers to how the body is able to repair an injury while maintaining the flow of blood to the rest of the circulatory system?
    (A) Coagulation
    (B) Vasoconstriction
    (C) Capillary exchange
    (D) Hemostasis

2. Discuss lifespan changes to the circulatory system

Fill in the Blank

1. While a fetus is in the womb, the ______________ circulatory system provides the fetus with oxygenated blood.
2. The foramen ovale and the ductus arteriosus must __________ for the newborn's heart to function properly.
3. As the heart matures and becomes more efficient, the heart rate gradually __________.
4. Changes of aging in the heart begin to occur as early as the late ______ and early ______.

Normal or Sign/Symptom

5. ____ Severe headache
6. ____ Heart pumps less efficiently in a geriatric patient
7. ____ Chest pain
8. ____ Swelling of hands or feet
9. ____ Pulse rate of 120 in an infant
10. ____ Bluish hands or feet
11. ____ Constant fatigue in a teenaged patient
12. ____ Shortness of breath

3. List common chronic and acute conditions of the circulatory system

Heart Disease

True or False

1. ____ Coronary artery disease (CAD) occurs when the coronary arteries widen and increase blood flow.
2. ____ CAD lowers the supply of blood, oxygen, and nutrients to the heart and can lead to heart attack or stroke.
3. ____ Angina is chest pain caused by reduced oxygen to the heart.
4. ____ The heart needs more oxygen when the body is at rest.
5. ____ Angina that occurs at rest or without stress is called *unstable angina*.
6. ____ A person with low cardiac output may have fatigue, a weak pulse, and low blood pressure.
7. ____ Cardiac arrest is rarely fatal.
8. ____ A stent is a small mesh tube placed against the walls of an artery to hold them open.
9. ____ Cardiomyopathy may cause the walls of the heart to dilate or to thicken.
10. ____ Left-sided congestive heart failure causes fluid buildup in the lungs.

Short Answer

11. What are three possible causes of hypertension?

____

____

____

____

____

12. Why is treatment of hypertension important?

____

____

____

____

____

13. How is hypertension treated?

____

____

____

____

Dysrhythmias

Fill in the Blank

14. Dysrhythmias, sometimes called ______________, are ______________ heart rhythms.

15. In the most life-threatening rhythms, ______________ fibrillation and ______________ fibrillation, the heart is fibrillating, or ______________.

16. Atrial fibrillation is especially common in ______________ patients. It can cause blood to ______________ in the heart.

17. Dysrhythmias are diagnosed by examining the patient and the patient's ______________.

Valvular Disorders/Inflammatory Disorders

Matching

Use each letter only once.

18. _____ Regurgitation
19. _____ Congenital defect
20. _____ Mitral valve prolapse
21. _____ Endocarditis
22. _____ Pericarditis

(A) A problem that occurred before birth; can be a cause of heart valve problems

(B) A potentially life-threatening condition in which the inner lining of the heart is inflamed

(C) Blood leaking back into the chamber from which it is being pumped; increases workload on the heart

(D) An inflammation of the membrane that surrounds the heart; in many cases the cause is unknown

(E) One example of heart valve disease; one or both of the valve flaps does not close properly

Vascular Diseases

Multiple Choice

23. Peripheral vascular disease is a condition in which the legs, feet, arms, or hands do not have enough
    (A) Cartilage
    (B) Fat
    (C) Blood circulation
    (D) Fluids

24. PVD is often caused by
    (A) Weakened bones
    (B) Weakened heart muscle due to damage
    (C) Infection of the lymph nodes
    (D) Fatty deposits in blood vessels

25. Varicose veins are caused by
    (A) Damaged valves in the veins
    (B) Ulcers of the legs and feet
    (C) Pathogens such as bacteria or fungi
    (D) Overuse of compression stockings

26. Which of these sets of conditions all relate to blood clots?
    (A) Hemophilia, aneurysm, and anemia
    (B) Thrombophlebitis, DVT, and pulmonary embolism
    (C) Aneurysm, anemia, and DVT
    (D) Hemophilia, thrombophilia, and anemia

27. Clots that block the arteries leading to the brain, or that travel to the brain, can cause a(n)
    (A) Myocardial infarction
    (B) Aneurysm
    (C) Dysrhythmia
    (D) Stroke

28. Pulmonary embolism is a dangerous risk associated with
    (A) Sickle cell disease
    (B) Coronary artery disease
    (C) Deep vein thrombosis
    (D) Superficial thrombophlebitis

Name: ______________________________

Blood Disorders

Fill in the Blank

29. The most common type of anemia is ____________________ anemia, caused by low __________ levels.

30. Treatment for anemia may include giving the patient oral or ______________________ iron, other medications, and/or ______________________ transfusions.

31. Instead of being disc-shaped, the red blood cells of a patient with sickle cell disease are shaped like a sickle, which is a(n) __________________ tool.

32. Deformed red blood cells in a patient with sickle cell disease can get __________ in blood vessels. This causes ____________ and can damage ____________.

33. Sickle cell disease is the most common _______________ blood condition in the US. As many as 1 in _______ Black Americans is born with SCD.

34. People with hemophilia are treated with infusions of the ______________________ _______ they lack.

35. People with thrombophilia may be treated with ______________________ medications.

36. Leukemia is a form of _______ in which the bone marrow produces defective ____________________ blood cells.

37. Leukemia can be treated with medications, chemotherapy, radiation, and ____________________ transplant.

38. Disorders of the blood are treated by ____________________.

4. Describe examinations and procedures related to the circulatory system

Short Answer

Place a check mark (✓) beside items below that may be part of a routine cardiology exam (not diagnostic procedures).

1. ____ Cardiac catheterization
2. ____ Auscultating heart sounds
3. ____ Examining the skin
4. ____ Stress test
5. ____ Echocardiography
6. ____ Checking vital signs
7. ____ Medication review
8. ____ Drawing blood for routine testing

Matching

Match each diagnostic procedure with a description below. Use each letter only once.

9. ____ Electrocardiography (EKG)
10. ____ Echocardiography
11. ____ Cardiac CT scanning
12. ____ Cardiac MRI
13. ____ Stress testing
14. ____ Cardiac catheterization

(A) Uses sound waves to produce images of blood flowing through the heart

(B) Uses a small tube threaded into the coronary arteries to check for blockages

(C) Uses electrocardiography to record the activity of the heart during exercise or when stimulated by medications

(D) Gives the provider a 3D image of the heart, coronary arteries, aorta, and pulmonary veins

(E) Shows all parts of the heart and can also show how blood moves in the heart

(F) A recording of the electrical activity of the heart

True or False

15. ____ MAs routinely perform echocardiograms.

16. ____ Some cardiologists perform stress testing at their offices.

17. ____ MAs can apply ambulatory monitors.

18. ____ Compression stockings may be ordered to treat cardiac dysrhythmias.

19. ____ When measuring a patient for thigh-high compression stockings, the MA measures the circumference of the thigh, the calf, and the length from the gluteal fold to the heel.

20. ____ Poorly fitted compression stockings are only a problem if they are uncomfortable.

5. Discuss patient education related to the circulatory system

Scenarios

1. Mimi is a 51-year-old patient whose weight and cholesterol levels have recently started to increase despite no change in her diet or activity level. Although she is generally active she does not have a regular exercise routine. Her doctor has suggested she start one and assigned Julia, an MA, to provide patient education about moderate aerobic exercise. What might Julia tell Mimi?

____

____

____

____

____

____

____

____

2. Hisham, age 62, regularly has blood pressure readings in the office that fall into the elevated range. His doctor does not want to begin medications yet, but wants him to monitor his blood pressure daily at home. What might June, the MA, be assigned to do?

____

____

____

____

____

3. Hisham's doctor also recommends a diet lower in sodium. What education could June provide about reducing sodium in Hisham's diet?

____

____

____

____

____

Short Answer

Write E *for signs and symptoms that may indicate a cardiac emergency. Write* P *for signs and symptoms that may indicate the development of heart disease and should be discussed with the provider.*

4. ____ Palpitations

5. ____ Pain that radiates, or extends down, one or both arms

6. ____ Swelling of the arms, hands, legs, or feet

7. ____ Sudden fatigue and weakness

8. ____ Changes in blood pressure

9. ____ Nausea along with a sensation of heavy pressure in the chest

10. ____ Racing heartbeat

Name: ______________________________

18

The Respiratory System and Related Care

1. Describe the structure and function of the respiratory system

True or False

1. ____ Respiration occurs in the lungs.
2. ____ Expiration is breathing in.
3. ____ The respiratory system brings oxygen into the body and eliminates carbon dioxide.
4. ____ The tonsils are made of lymphatic tissue.
5. ____ The vocal cords are located in the trachea.
6. ____ The larynx is also called the windpipe.
7. ____ Oxygen and carbon dioxide are exchanged between the alveoli and the capillaries.
8. ____ The pleura is a two-layered membrane that covers the lungs.

Multiple Choice

9. The lower trachea divides into two branches called
   (A) Alveoli
   (B) Bronchi
   (C) Tonsils
   (D) The nasopharynx and the oropharynx
10. The three forms of respiration are
   (A) Shallow, deep, and rapid
   (B) External, internal, and cellular
   (C) Distal, medial, and proximal
   (D) Acidic, alkaline, and neutral
11. Which of the following is true?
   (A) Both lungs are the same size.
   (B) The left lung is slightly larger than the right lung.
   (C) The left lung is twice as large as the right lung.
   (D) The right lung is slightly larger than the left lung.
12. What is located between the layers of the pleura?
   (A) The alveoli
   (B) Lubricating fluid
   (C) The pulmonary arteries
   (D) Lymphatic tissue that protects the respiratory system from pathogens

2. Discuss lifespan changes to the respiratory system

Fill in the Blank

1. The lungs begin to function ________ birth.
2. A newborn's airway is filled with ____________.
3. Lung capacity increases throughout childhood as more ______________ are formed in the lungs.
4. The lungs become fully mature around ___________ year(s) of age.
5. As an adult reaches their _______________ lung capacity starts to decrease.

Normal or Sign/Symptom

6. ____ In a pediatric patient, shortness of breath after walking a short distance

7. ____ Oxygen saturation of 99%
8. ____ Rattling sound heard when auscultating the lungs
9. ____ A weak voice in a patient who is 82 years old
10. ____ Decreased ability to exercise intensely in a patient who is 55 years old
11. ____ Bluish tint to the nail beds

3. List common chronic and acute conditions of the respiratory system

Short Answer

1. Describe three types of healthcare workers who care for patients with respiratory conditions.

____

____

____

____

____

____

____

____

2. Why are antibiotics not prescribed for viral infections?

____

____

____

____

3. In what situations might a provider not prescribe an antibiotic for a bacterial infection?

____

____

____

____

Conditions Affecting the Upper and/or Lower Respiratory Tracts

Matching

Use each letter only once.

4. ____ Rhinitis
5. ____ Sinusitis
6. ____ Upper respiratory infection
7. ____ Tonsillitis
8. ____ Strep throat
9. ____ Laryngitis
10. ____ Obstructive sleep apnea
11. ____ Influenza
12. ____ COVID-19

(A) Commonly called a cold; usually results from a viral infection of the nose, sinuses, and throat

(B) A viral respiratory illness that is especially common in the fall and winter; different strains spread each year

(C) Inflammation of the linings of the sinuses

(D) Infection of the tonsils/throat by the bacterium *Streptococcus pyogenes*

(E) Inflammation of the mucous membranes lining the nasal passages

(F) A breathing disorder in which a person repeatedly stops breathing during sleep

(G) A viral respiratory illness spread by droplets and airborne viral particles; enclosed spaces with poor ventilation increase the risk of infection

(H) Inflammation of the tonsils; caused by viral or bacterial infections

(I) Inflammation of the larynx; may be caused by infection, irritation, or overuse of the voice

Conditions Affecting the Lungs

Multiple Choice

13. Which of the following is true of pneumonia?
    (A) It is always caused by bacteria.
    (B) It is always caused by a virus.
    (C) It may be caused by a bacterial, viral, or fungal infection.
    (D) Recovery is faster for older adults.

14. Which of the following is a symptom of pleurisy?
    (A) Nasal congestion
    (B) Chest pain that becomes worse with breathing
    (C) Loss of the senses of taste and smell
    (D) Brain fog/disorientation

15. This is an occupational disease associated with workers who have high exposure to dusts:
    (A) COPD
    (B) Emphysema
    (C) Pleurisy
    (D) Pneumoconiosis

16. These are the two chronic lung diseases grouped under COPD:
    (A) Asthma and bronchitis
    (B) Emphysema and chronic pneumonia
    (C) Chronic bronchitis and emphysema
    (D) Pneumoconiosis and bronchiectasis

17. Orthopnea, or difficulty breathing when lying down that is relieved by sitting up, is a common symptom of
    (A) Asthma
    (B) COPD
    (C) Pneumonia
    (D) Lung cancer

18. Bronchitis is usually caused by
    (A) Bacteria
    (B) Exposure to cold weather
    (C) Environmental toxins
    (D) A virus

19. Two types of tuberculosis are
    (A) Chronic and acute
    (B) Pulmonary and cardiac
    (C) Latent TB infection and TB disease
    (D) Contagious and non-contagious

20. Who is more likely to get TB?
    (A) People with weakened immune systems
    (B) People who had chickenpox as children
    (C) People who have not been vaccinated against it
    (D) People who do not get adequate exercise

21. Postural drainage, which involves using different body positions to drain mucus from the lungs or to loosen it so it can be coughed up, may be ordered for a patient with this condition:
    (A) Influenza
    (B) Lung cancer
    (C) Bronchiectasis
    (D) Bronchitis

22. What causes the coughing and wheezing that occurs with asthma?
    (A) Air trapped in the lungs by constricted, mucus-filled airways
    (B) Spasms in the trachea (windpipe)
    (C) Abnormally enlarged bronchial tubes
    (D) Fluid in the lungs that interferes with gas exchange

Short Answer

For each of the following conditions, list at least three signs/symptoms, the etiology (cause), and at least one form of treatment.

23. Emphysema

Signs/symptoms: ______________________________

____

____

____

Etiology: ______________________________

____

____

Treatment: ______________________________

____

____

Name: ______________________

24. Asthma

Signs/symptoms: ______________________

Etiology: ______________________

Treatment: ______________________

25. Lung cancer

Signs/symptoms: ______________________

Etiology: ______________________

Treatment: ______________________

26. Pulmonary edema

Signs/symptoms: ______________________

Etiology: ______________________

Treatment: ______________________

27. Acute respiratory distress syndrome (ARDS)

Signs/symptoms: ______________________

Etiology: ______________________

Treatment: ______________________

28. Respiratory failure

Signs/symptoms: ______________________

Etiology: ______________________

Treatment: ______________________

29. Infant respiratory distress syndrome (hyaline membrane disease)

Signs/symptoms: ______________________

Name: ______________________________

Etiology: ______________________________

____

____

Treatment: ______________________________

____

____

4. Describe examinations and procedures related to the respiratory system

Short Answer

Place a check mark (✓) beside items below that may be part of a routine respiratory examination.

1. _____ Auscultating lung sounds
2. _____ A 6-minute walking test
3. _____ A treadmill stress test
4. _____ A sweat chloride test
5. _____ Observing for respiratory effort
6. _____ Measurement of arterial blood gases
7. _____ Observing the skin
8. _____ Pulmonary function tests

Matching

Use each letter only once.

9. _____ Residual volume
10. _____ Crackles/rales
11. _____ Tidal volume
12. _____ Peak expiratory flow rate (PEFR)
13. _____ Total lung capacity
14. _____ Wheezes
15. _____ Forced vital capacity
16. _____ Rhonchi
17. _____ Vital capacity

(A) The maximum amount of air a person can inhale

(B) The amount of air that remains in the lungs after the patient has exhaled

(C) High-pitched, whistling sounds that occur most often during expiration

(D) The amount of air that a person can exhale slowly after inhaling as much as possible

(E) Rattling sounds that are heard during inspiration

(F) The amount of air that flows into and leaves the lungs during respirations

(G) The maximum amount of air that a person can exhale quickly and forcefully after inhaling as much as possible

(H) Low-pitched, snoring sounds that are heard on expiration

(I) The maximum speed at which a person can exhale air from the lungs

True or False

18. _____ Most providers prefer that patients not smoke for at least 24 hours before having pulmonary function tests.
19. _____ Pulmonary function tests must be repeated until five acceptable measurements are obtained.
20. _____ During pulmonary function tests the patient can choose whether to breathe through their mouth or their nose.
21. _____ A peak flow meter measures total lung capacity.
22. _____ An asthma patient whose PEFR is in the red zone should use their inhaler and report the readings to the provider.
23. _____ An asthma patient whose PEFR is in the yellow zone has a PEFR that is 50%–80% of their personal best reading.
24. _____ When assisting with the use of a peak flow meter, the MA should consider the highest of three readings to be the patient's PEFR.
25. _____ A spacer is an attachment that filters out some of the medication from a metered dose inhaler, lowering the dose for a pediatric patient.

Name: ______________________________

26. ____ Patients with asthma or other chronic respiratory conditions may have a nebulizer at home for self-administered treatments.

27. ____ Oxygen therapy must be ordered by a provider and the dosage must be specified.

28. ____ Breathing tubes may be inserted via a gastrostomy.

Fill in the Blank

29. The ________________ and ________________ may be swabbed and tested for pathogens including strep, influenza, mononucleosis, and ________________.

30. Nasopharyngeal swabs have ________________ applicators to make it easier to access the nasopharynx.

31. Allow children to sit in a(n) ________________ during a swabbing procedure if they wish to do so.

32. When swabbing the throat do not touch the patient's ________________. This can cause a(n) ______ reflex.

33. When performing a nasopharyngeal swab, it is important not to ________________ any obstructions. This may ____________ the patient.

34. It is easiest to collect sputum ________________ in the morning, if possible.

35. Proper PPE for collecting a sputum specimen includes gloves and a(n) ________________ or similar respirator.

5. Discuss patient education related to the respiratory system

Scenarios

1. Pedro is an 85-year-old in good health, but he is concerned about contracting COVID-19, influenza, and other respiratory illnesses during the fall and winter. His doctor asks MA Kayden to provide Pedro with information about respiratory hygiene and steps he can take to avoid respiratory illnesses. What might Kayden discuss with Pedro?

____

2. Sheridan, a 2-year-old, is at her pediatrician's office for a well check. The doctor asks MA Joaquin to review information about choking hazards with Sheridan's grandfather, who brought her to the appointment. What information should Joaquin include?

____

Name: ______________________________

____

____

____

____

____

____

____

3. Delbert is a 78-year-old who has recently been diagnosed with sleep apnea. His doctor prescribed a CPAP machine and Delbert reports that he has the machine. MA Charlene is assigned to review instructions for care and use with him. What should she cover during their talk?

____

____

____

____

____

____

____

____

____

____

____

____

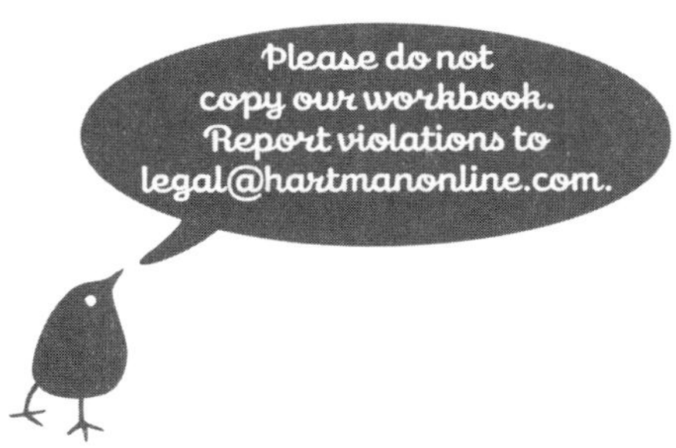

Name: ______________________________

Name: ____________________

19

The Urinary System and Related Care

1. Describe the structure and function of the urinary system

Short Answer

1. What are the parts of the urinary system?

____

____

2. What happens when blood flows through the kidneys?

____

____

3. What is one reason why the female bladder is more likely to become infected by bacteria than the male bladder?

____

____

4. Where is the renal medulla located within the kidney?

____

____

5. What are the functional units of the kidney that filter blood?

____

____

6. How is the urge to urinate triggered?

____

____

7. What are the two substances the kidneys secrete that are vital to homeostasis? What does each substance do?

____

____

____

____

____

2. Discuss lifespan changes to the urinary system

Fill in the Blank

1. The kidneys begin to function _______________, but they are not fully _______________.
2. A newborn baby's kidneys cannot retain _______________ efficiently, making _______________ a risk for infants.
3. Most children develop full bladder control at around _______________ years of age.
4. The rate at which blood is filtered by the kidneys is called the _______________ filtration rate.
5. A healthy person has a GFR of _______________ per minute or more. The GFR gradually _______________ with age.
6. Older adults, like infants, have a higher risk of _______________.

Normal or Sign/Symptom

7. ____ Pain during urination
8. ____ Patient who is middle-aged has to get up at night to urinate
9. ____ Bladder always feels full or painful
10. ____ Pain in kidney region
11. ____ Urinary incontinence in patient who is elderly
12. ____ Dehydration

3. List common chronic and acute conditions of the urinary system

Fill in the Blank

1. ________________ diagnose and treat kidney disorders such as kidney failure.
2. ________________ treat disorders of the bladder and urethra. They also specialize in care for the ________________ ________________ system.
3. A(n) ________________ treats female urinary system disorders.

Inflammation and Infection

True or False

4. ____ Urinary tract infections are more common in men than in women.
5. ____ When a person has a UTI, she may experience a painful burning sensation during urination.
6. ____ Poor fluid intake and holding urine in for long periods can contribute to UTIs.
7. ____ *Pyelonephritis* is the medical term for inflammation of the bladder.
8. ____ A UTI can lead to sepsis, a life-threatening condition caused by the body's response to an infection.
9. ____ The signs and symptoms of interstitial cystitis can mimic a UTI.
10. ____ Interstitial cystitis causes chronic inflammation of the kidneys.

Urinary Flow Disorders

Multiple Choice

11. Which of the following is true of urinary incontinence?
    (A) It is more common in young adults than in other patients.
    (B) There is only one form of urinary incontinence.
    (C) Treatment usually involves surgery.
    (D) It is not a normal part of aging.
12. What type of exercise can help prevent urinary incontinence in women?
    (A) Weight-bearing
    (B) Aerobic
    (C) Pelvic floor strengthening
    (D) Endurance-building
13. In what patient population is urinary retention more common?
    (A) Infants and toddlers
    (B) Men
    (C) Women
    (D) Pregnant women
14. A kidney stone that cannot be passed may lead to urinary obstruction and this condition:
    (A) Hydronephrosis
    (B) Urinary incontinence
    (C) Neurogenic bladder
    (D) Interstitial cystitis
15. Neurogenic bladder may require this procedure:
    (A) Lithotripsy
    (B) Biopsy
    (C) Intermittent catheterization
    (D) Placement of an indwelling catheter

Conditions of the Kidneys

Fill in the Blank

16. Signs and symptoms of kidney stones may not be noticeable until the stones begin to move down the ________________, causing pain.
17. Lithotripsy is a procedure that uses ________________ to break up kidney stones.

18. People with polycystic kidney disease are at high risk for developing ______________.

19. Pyelonephritis is an acute, ______________ infection of the kidney.

20. Acute glomerulonephritis may be caused by a(n) ______________ infection such as strep throat.

21. Chronic glomerulonephritis is often ______________ and may cause complete kidney failure.

22. Renovascular ______________ is a condition in which a blockage of arteries in the kidneys causes high blood pressure

23. People with chronic kidney disease have a reduced glomerular filtration rate of ______________ mL/minute.

24. ______________ is an artificial means of removing the body's waste products.

25. Chronic renal failure can progress to end-stage renal disease. This is fatal without kidney dialysis or a kidney ______________.

Other Disorders of the Kidneys and Bladder

Short Answer

For the conditions in questions 26 and 27, list at least three signs/symptoms, the etiology (cause), and at least one form of treatment.

26. Cystocele

Signs/symptoms: ______________

Etiology: ______________

Treatment: ______________

27. Renal cell cancer

Signs/symptoms: ______________

Etiology: ______________

Treatment: ______________

28. What are three risk factors for developing bladder cancer?

29. What has happened in Stage IV cancer?

30. How are some chemotherapy medications administered for bladder cancer?

Name: ____________________

4. Describe examinations and procedures related to the urinary system

Matching

Use each letter only once.

1. ____ 24-hour urine specimen
2. ____ Clean-catch specimen
3. ____ First void specimen
4. ____ Culture and sensitivity test
5. ____ Routine urine specimen
6. ____ Suprapubic aspiration

(A) A test that can identify microorganisms in the urine; ordered if a patient has had repeated or severe UTIs

(B) Urine sample collected any time a patient voids

(C) Also called *midstream* specimen

(D) Procedure for collecting a urine specimen using a needle inserted through the abdomen

(E) Collects all urine voided in 24 hours

(F) Urine specimen that is collected when the patient first urinates in the morning

Multiple Choice

7. One type of reagent (dip) strip test measures how acidic or alkaline urine is; it measures the ________.
   (A) Food
   (B) pH level
   (C) Illegal drugs
   (D) Fat

8. The presence of glucose or ketones in urine may be a sign of
   (A) High blood pressure
   (B) Thyroid disorder
   (C) Anemia
   (D) Diabetes

9. Occult blood in urine is
   (A) A normal change of aging
   (B) Easily seen
   (C) Hidden
   (D) A sign of anemia

10. A urine specific gravity test
    (A) Checks for adequate oxygen levels
    (B) Indicates the specific type of urinary incontinence a patient is experiencing
    (C) Counts the amount of blood cells in urine
    (D) Shows how the density of urine compares to the density of water

11. A double-voided urine specimen may be used to test for
    (A) Glucose
    (B) Sweat
    (C) Sputum
    (D) Nitrites

12. Which of the following may be done when collecting a urine specimen for drug testing?
    (A) The MA may accompany the patient into the bathroom.
    (B) Coloring may be added to the toilet water.
    (C) The patient may be asked to take a polygraph test.
    (D) The patient may be asked to take an oath of honesty.

13. When preparing a patient for a 24-hour collection, what equipment is often sent home with the patient?
    (A) Test tubes holding chemical agents the patient must add to the specimen
    (B) A collection bag with adhesive that is fitted over the genitals
    (C) Wipes for cleaning the genital area before each void
    (D) A hat for the toilet and/or a urinal

5. Discuss patient education related to the urinary system

Scenarios

1. Esther is 58 and has been experiencing occasional stress incontinence. Alina has been assigned to instruct Esther about exercises to strengthen her pelvic floor muscles. What should Alina tell Esther?

2. Gianna is 23. She has had four UTIs over the past year. During her annual gynecological exam she asks if there is anything she can do to prevent these infections. The doctor asks her MA, Camila, to review UTI prevention with Gianna. What topics should Camila cover?

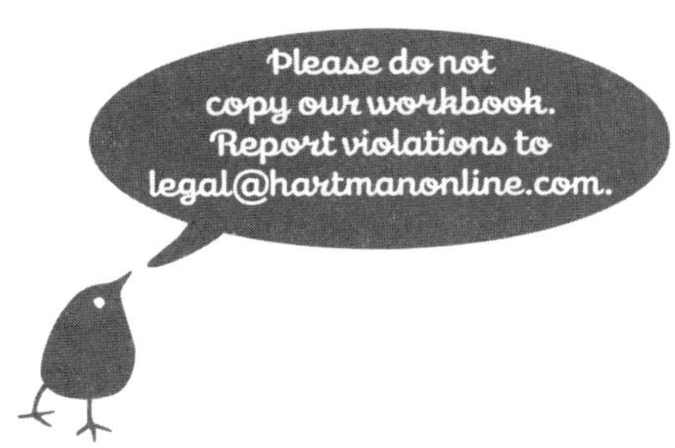

Name: ______________________________

Name: ______________________________

20

The Gastrointestinal System and Related Care

1. Describe the structure and function of the gastrointestinal system

Crossword

Across

3. Process of expelling wastes (made up of the waste products of food and fluids) that are not absorbed into the cells
4. Involuntary contractions that move food into the stomach from the esophagus
6. Transfer of nutrients from the intestines to the cells
7. Semisolid material made up of water, solid waste material, bacteria, and mucus that passes through the rectum and out of the body

Down

1. Process of preparing food physically and chemically so that it can be absorbed into the cells
2. Semiliquid substance created by the breaking down of food in the stomach
5. Muscular pouch located in the upper left part of the abdominal cavity

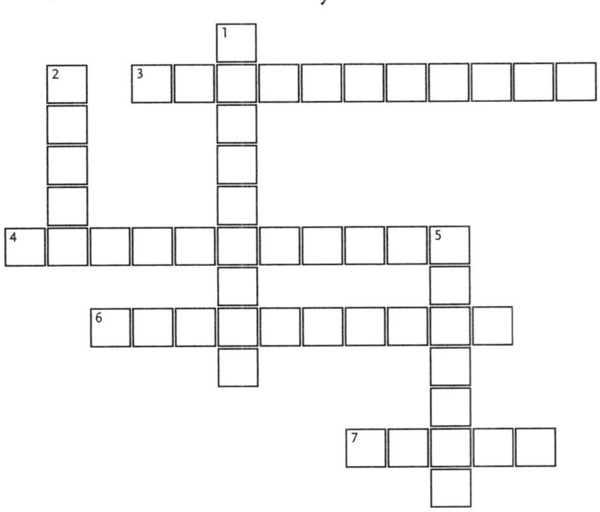

Matching

Use each letter only once.

8. _____ Maxillary teeth
9. _____ Mandibular teeth
10. _____ Dental caries
11. _____ Gingivae
12. _____ Incisors
13. _____ Cuspids
14. _____ Bicuspids
15. _____ Molars

(A) Tooth decay

(B) Teeth that tear tough food

(C) Upper teeth

(D) Connective tissue that protects the roots of the teeth

(E) The strongest and most numerous teeth

(F) Teeth that bite into food

(G) Teeth that grind and smash food into smaller pieces

(H) Lower teeth

2. Discuss lifespan changes to the gastrointestinal system

Fill in the Blank

1. In the uterus, the fetus swallows ______________ fluid.
2. Some material builds up in the fetus's intestines. It is called ______________ and it is eliminated in the first ______________ soon after birth.

Name: ______________________________

3. By approximately ______________________, the digestive system produces the enzymes necessary to digest proteins and fats. At this time ________________ foods may be introduced.

4. Most providers recommend that babies continue to receive breast milk or formula until at least ________ of age.

5. By late ______________________, the digestive tract has reached maturity and remains fully functional in early and middle adulthood.

Normal or Sign/Symptom

6. ____ Difficulty recognizing/describing gastrointestinal symptoms (young child)

7. ____ Frequent diarrhea

8. ____ Bloating and flatulence after every meal

9. ____ Increased constipation in a patient who is middle-aged

10. ____ Complete loss of sense of taste

11. ____ Slow chewing and swallowing in a patient who is elderly

12. ____ Heartburn

3. List common chronic and acute conditions of the gastrointestinal system

True or False

1. ____ A gastroenterologist focuses specifically on disorders of the stomach.

2. ____ *Proctologist* and *colorectal surgeon* are two terms for the same type of medical specialist.

3. ____ A colorectal surgeon specializes in surgery for weight loss.

4. ____ A hepatologist treats diseases and disorders of the liver and accessory digestive organs.

5. ____ Dentists care for the teeth, gums, and oral cavity.

Nausea, Vomiting, Diarrhea, and Gastroenteritis/Upper Gastrointestinal Tract Conditions

Multiple Choice

6. This condition is often referred to as the *stomach flu*, although it is not caused by the influenza virus.
(A) Gastritis
(B) Gastroenteritis
(C) Gastric ulcers
(D) Gastroesophageal reflux disease

7. These may be caused by excessive acid secretion or by a bacterium called *H. pylori*:
(A) Nausea and vomiting
(B) Diarrhea and dehydration
(C) Peptic ulcers
(D) Heartburn and constipation

8. This is the most common symptom of gastroesophageal reflux disease (GERD):
(A) Heartburn
(B) Diarrhea
(C) Nausea
(D) Vomiting

9. Drugs used to treat peptic ulcers and GERD are also used to treat
(A) Gastroenteritis
(B) Hiatal hernia
(C) Gastritis
(D) Hemorrhoids

Obesity

Short Answer

10. List four factors that may contribute to obesity.

____

____

____

____

____

____

11. What is the benefit of treating obesity?

____

____

____

____

____

12. List one obesity myth you are familiar with. What is a more accurate understanding?

____

____

____

____

____

____

Gastrointestinal System Hernias

Short Answer

For each item, mark H *for hiatal hernia or* I *for inguinal hernia.*

13. ____ A portion of the small intestine protrudes.
14. ____ Eating small, frequent meals can help.
15. ____ An endoscopy may be performed to check for tissue damage in the esophagus.
16. ____ Can become life-threatening if blood flow to the intestines is cut off
17. ____ Most hernias of this type require surgery.

Constipation and Hemorrhoids

Fill in the Blank

18. Constipation occurs when the feces move too ____________ through the intestine.
19. Treatment for constipation includes increasing the amount of ______________ eaten and ____________ consumed and increasing ____________ level.
20. Medications called ____________ may be ordered for constipation.
21. A fecal ______________ is a hard stool that is stuck in the rectum and cannot be expelled.
22. Early assessment of ______________ may help prevent impactions.
23. Rectal ______________, burning, pain, and ______________ during bowel elimination are signs and symptoms of hemorrhoids.
24. Chronic constipation, obesity, pregnancy, chronic diarrhea, overuse of ______________ and enemas, and ______________ during bowel movements are common causes of hemorrhoids.

Chronic Bowel Conditions

Matching

Use each letter only once.

25. ____ Irritable bowel syndrome (IBS)
26. ____ Inflammatory bowel disease (IBD)
27. ____ Ulcerative colitis
28. ____ Crohn's disease
29. ____ Diverticulosis
30. ____ Diverticulitis

(A) Functional condition that results from problems in communication between the nervous system and the digestive tract

(B) A condition in which small pouches in the colon *diverticula* become inflamed

(C) Most commonly affects the small intestine; may occur in patches, with damaged tissue among healthy tissue

(D) Chronic inflammatory disease of the large intestine; can cause intestinal bleeding and death if left untreated

(E) A term for conditions in which the bowel is chronically inflamed; thought to be caused by improper immune system response

(F) The development of small pouches called *diverticula* in the colon

Name: ____________________

Cancers of the Gastrointestinal System

Short Answer

For each of the following forms of cancer, list either two risk factors or two signs/symptoms, as indicated.

31. Oral cancer

Risk factors: ____________________

____

____

32. Esophageal cancer

Risk factors: ____________________

____

____

33. Gastric cancer

Signs/symptoms: ____________________

____

____

34. Pancreatic cancer

Risk factors: ____________________

____

____

35. Colorectal cancer

Signs/symptoms: ____________________

____

____

Conditions of the Liver, Gallbladder, and Pancreas

True or False

36. ____ The most common types of hepatitis are hepatitis C, D, and E.

37. ____ Cholelithiasis is a condition in which small stones form in the kidneys.

38. ____ Cirrhosis is a disease in which liver tissue has been replaced by scar tissue.

39. ____ High triglycerides, alcoholism, injury, gallstones, and pancreatic cancer can all cause pancreatitis.

40. ____ Hepatitis and chronic alcoholism are common causes of cholecystitis.

4. Describe examinations and procedures related to the gastrointestinal system

Short Answer

1. List three techniques the provider may use when examining a patient's gastrointestinal system.

____

____

____

____

2. What are four things a stool sample may be tested for?

____

____

____

____

3. Briefly describe the two types of fecal occult blood testing.

____

____

____

____

____

____

____

____

____

____

____

____

4. List four items that patients are asked not to consume before and during fecal guaiac testing.

____

____

____

____

5. What three things should patients be asked not to include in a stool sample?

____

____

____

6. List four conditions that may be diagnosed during a barium study.

____

____

____

____

7. What three steps may an MA instruct a patient about before a colonoscopy?

____

____

____

____

____

____

____

____

____

____

5. Discuss patient education related to the gastrointestinal system

Short Answer

Write the letter of the correct nutrient beside each description below. Use a W *for water,* C *for carbohydrates,* P *for proteins,* F *for fats,* V *for vitamins, and* M *for minerals. Letters may be used more than once.*

1. ____ Sources include seafood, beans, poultry, and vegetarian meat substitutes.
2. ____ A person can only survive a few days without this.
3. ____ These build bones and help in blood formation.
4. ____ These add flavor to food and help to absorb certain vitamins.
5. ____ They are essential for maintaining muscle strength.
6. ____ Saturated and trans types can increase cholesterol levels and the risk of some diseases.
7. ____ The body cannot make most of these nutrients; they must be obtained by eating certain foods.
8. ____ Simple ones do not have the same nutritional value as complex ones.
9. ____ Examples include bread, cereal, and potatoes.
10. ____ This is the most essential nutrient for life.
11. ____ Categories include monounsaturated and polyunsaturated.
12. ____ This is needed by every cell in the body.
13. ____ These can be fat-soluble or water-soluble.
14. ____ These help the body store energy.
15. ____ Iron and calcium are examples.

Name: ______________________________

Short Answer

The USDA developed the MyPlate icon and website to promote healthy eating practices. Looking at the MyPlate icon, fill in the food groups.

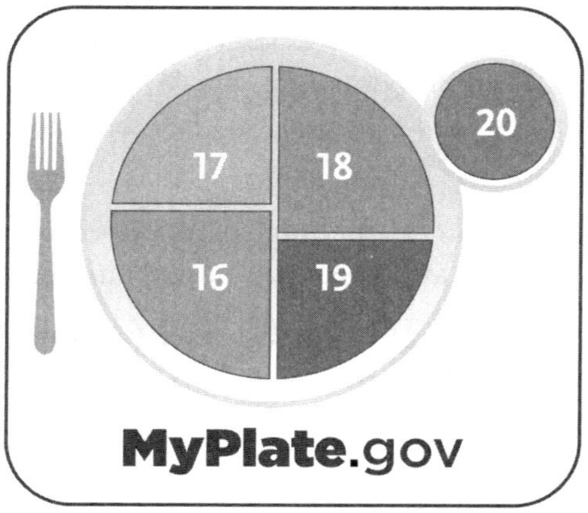

16. ______________________________
17. ______________________________
18. ______________________________
19. ______________________________
20. ______________________________
21. Describe the last meal you ate. Organize the food into the MyPlate food groups and give an estimate of how much of each food group made up your plate.

Multiple Choice

22. According to MyPlate, half of a person's plate should be made up of
    (A) Grains and protein
    (B) Vegetables and fruits
    (C) Seafood and dairy
    (D) Grains and dairy
23. Which of the following is a plant-based protein?
    (A) Salmon
    (B) Eggs
    (C) Sausage
    (D) Beans
24. Most dairy group choices should be
    (A) Full fat
    (B) 2% fat at most
    (C) Half-and-half
    (D) 1% fat at most
25. Which of the following foods is considered high in sodium?
    (A) Apple
    (B) Pickle
    (C) Avocado
    (D) Corn on the cob

Scenarios

26. At Joni's 8-year well check her mother tells the doctor that Joni could use some encouragement in oral hygiene habits. MA Isabel is asked to review oral hygiene guidelines with Joni. What should she mention?

27. Ignacio has just had a colostomy. The pouching system he uses has preattached wafers. MA Michaela is assigned to review ostomy care with Ignacio. What information should she include?

Name: ______________________

21

The Endocrine System and Related Care

1. Describe the structure and function of the endocrine system

Matching

Use each letter only once.

1. ____ Adrenal glands
2. ____ Antidiuretic hormone
3. ____ Gonads
4. ____ Insulin
5. ____ Oxytocin
6. ____ Pancreas
7. ____ Parathyroid glands
8. ____ Pituitary gland
9. ____ Thyroid gland
10. ____ Follicle-stimulating hormone
11. ____ Luteinizing hormone
12. ____ Thymus gland
13. ____ Adrenaline
14. ____ Glucocorticoids

(A) Secretes insulin

(B) Produce hormones that regulate salt and water absorption in kidneys and produce the hormone adrenaline

(C) Located in the neck in front of the larynx and produces thyroid hormone

(D) Secretes key hormones that stimulate the rest of the body's endocrine glands

(E) Secretes a hormone to regulate calcium use

(F) Moves glucose from the blood into the cells for energy for the body

(G) Controls the balance of fluids in the body

(H) Causes the uterus to contract during and after childbirth

(I) Produces hormones that regulate the ability to reproduce

(J) Released by the adrenal glands; help regulate metabolism

(K) Secretes hormones that regulate the production of T cells

(L) Closely tied to the body's "fight or flight" response to perceived threats

(M) In the female, stimulates estrogen production; in the male, stimulates sperm production

(N) Stimulates ovulation in females and testosterone production in males

2. Discuss lifespan changes to the endocrine system

Fill in the Blank

1. The endocrine system begins to release hormones into the bloodstream ____________ birth.
2. Hormone production is necessary for normal ______________ and ________________ during childhood.
3. At birth, the ______________ gland is the most fully developed of the endocrine glands, helping to protect the infant from ______________ during this very vulnerable stage of life.
4. The thymus gland begins to ______________ with age.

Name: ____________________

5. During puberty, the ______________ gland stimulates the gonads to produce hormones that control the development of ______________ sex characteristics.

6. Puberty continues through the ________________ years until full maturity is reached in ____________ adulthood.

7. ________________ hormone is necessary for normal development in childhood and for maintaining the health of body tissues in ________________.

Normal or Sign/System

8. ____ No signs of puberty in a 16-year-old girl

9. ____ Decreased thymus activity in an adult

10. ____ Rapid growth in a 13-year-old patient

11. ____ Lower metabolism in a middle-aged patient

12. ____ Very short stature and lack of expected growth in a 10-year-old patient

13. ____ Irregular menstrual periods and other signs of lower estrogen levels in a 50-year-old female patient

3. List common chronic and acute conditions of the endocrine system

Pituitary Gland Disorders

Short Answer

1. Undersecretion of which hormone is a common cause of dwarfism?

____

2. What is the difference between gigantism and acromegaly?

____

____

____

____

3. Which two conditions described in the textbook relate to the secretion of antidiuretic hormone (ADH)? For each condition, state whether ADH is oversecreted or undersecreted.

____

____

____

____

Thyroid/Parathyroid Disorders

True or False

4. ____ Graves' disease is an autoimmune disorder that often causes hyperthyroidism.

5. ____ Hyperthyroidism causes slower metabolism, fatigue, and cold intolerance.

6. ____ Congenital hypothyroidism is most commonly caused by iodine deficiency during pregnancy.

7. ____ Treatment of hyperthyroidism may include surgical removal of part of the thyroid.

8. ____ Thyroid storm is caused by a rapid rise in thyroid levels.

9. ____ Hashimoto's thyroiditis is an autoimmune disorder that often causes hypothyroidism.

10. ____ Myxedema is a complication of untreated hypothyroidism that affects patients in middle age and older.

11. ____ Low calcium levels in the blood may be a sign of hyperparathyroidism.

12. ____ Parathyroid disease can cause irregular heartbeats and weakened bones.

Pancreatic Disorders

Multiple Choice

13. Diabetes is a condition in which the pancreas does not produce any or enough, or does not properly use
    (A) Insulin
    (B) Glucose
    (C) Growth hormones
    (D) Adrenaline

14. Sugars collecting in the blood cause problems with
    (A) Breathing
    (B) Circulation
    (C) Pain level
    (D) Ambulation

15. Type 1 diabetes
    (A) Continues throughout a person's life
    (B) Is most common in the elderly
    (C) Is first treated with surgery
    (D) Does not require a change of diet

16. Changes in the circulatory system from diabetes can cause
    (A) Hair loss
    (B) Heart attack and stroke
    (C) Multiple sclerosis
    (D) COPD

17. The most common form of diabetes is
    (A) Insulin reaction
    (B) Gestational diabetes
    (C) Type 1 diabetes
    (D) Type 2 diabetes

18. Poor circulation and impaired wound healing may result in
    (A) Urinary tract infections
    (B) Cancer
    (C) Leg and foot ulcers
    (D) An autoimmune disease

19. Gangrene can lead to
    (A) Loss of bowel control
    (B) Peripheral vascular disease
    (C) Congestive heart failure
    (D) Amputation

20. What condition occurs when a person's blood glucose level is above normal but not high enough for a diagnosis of type 2 diabetes?
    (A) Gestational diabetes
    (B) Type 1 diabetes
    (C) Prediabetes
    (D) Hyperglycemia

21. One sign of diabetes is peripheral neuropathy, a form of nerve damage that causes
    (A) Tingling or numbness in hands or feet
    (B) Loss of bladder control
    (C) Bowel dysfunction
    (D) Shooting pains from the buttocks down the back of the leg

22. Which of the following is a physiological reason why diabetes may be challenging to control during adolescence?
    (A) Adolescents do not like to follow instructions.
    (B) Dramatic changes are occurring in the body.
    (C) Adolescents often have an unhealthy diet.
    (D) Adolescents may not get enough exercise.

23. What medical specialist treats diabetes and other endocrine disorders?
    (A) An endocrinologist
    (B) A urologist
    (C) A diabetologist
    (D) A hormonologist

Adrenal Disorders

Short Answer

For each of the following conditions, list at least three signs/symptoms and the etiology (cause) of the disease.

24. Addison's disease

Signs/symptoms: ______________________

____

____

____

Name: ______________________

Etiology: ______________________

____

____

25. Cushing disease

Signs/symptoms: ______________________

____

____

____

Etiology: ______________________

____

____

4. Describe examinations and procedures related to the endocrine system

Fill in the Blank

1. The provider may order a variety of ______________ and ______________ tests to check endocrine function.
2. There are several types of ______________ glucose tests.
3. A specimen for a(n) ______________ blood sugar test must be taken when the patient has not eaten or drunk anything (other than water) within the past ______________ hours.
4. Oral glucose challenge tests and oral glucose tolerance tests are often used to screen for ______________.
5. Hemoglobin A1c tests measure average blood glucose levels over a period of several ______________.
6. Results of hemoglobin A1c can show how well a patient's ______________ is managed.
7. ______________ is one form of diagnostic imaging that can be performed in the office during a routine patient visit.
8. ______________ is one of the most common hormones administered in the medical office.
9. A biopsy performed by inserting a needle and aspirating material, or drawing material into a syringe, is called a(n) ______________ biopsy.

5. Discuss patient education related to the endocrine system

Scenarios

1. Haylee is a freshman in college and has been having difficulty managing her type 1 diabetes. Her endocrinologist has referred her to a dietitian to help manage her nutrition. He has also asked MA Robin to review with Haylee tips for getting better sleep. What should Robin mention?

____

____

____

____

____

____

____

____

____

____

____

____

____

____

____

Name: ______________________

2. What are some of the basic guidelines that are likely to be part of the dietitian's plan for Haylee?

Name: ______________________________

22

The Reproductive System and Related Care

1. Describe the structure and function of the reproductive system

Multiple Choice

1. The reproductive system allows humans to
   (A) Move and speak
   (B) Create human life
   (C) Think logically
   (D) Fight disease

2. The hormone needed for male reproductive organs to function properly is
   (A) Sperm
   (B) Adrenaline
   (C) Estrogen
   (D) Testosterone

3. The male and female sex glands are the
   (A) Glands
   (B) Ureters
   (C) Gonads
   (D) Urethras

4. The tube through which males pass both urine and semen is called the
   (A) Prostate
   (B) Penis
   (C) Urethra
   (D) Seminal vesicle

5. The gonads in human females are called
   (A) Ovaries
   (B) Eggs
   (C) Testicles
   (D) Sex cells

6. The female reproductive cycle is maintained by the hormones
   (A) Estrogen and progesterone
   (B) Adrenaline and progesterone
   (C) Testosterone and ADH
   (D) Insulin and testosterone

7. Luteinizing hormone and follicle-stimulating hormone are involved in triggering
   (A) Menstrual bleeding
   (B) Development of secondary sex characteristics
   (C) Ovulation
   (D) The release of milk for a newborn baby

8. The ________ contains blood vessels to provide for the growth of an embryo.
   (A) Endometrium
   (B) Uterus
   (C) Fallopian tube
   (D) Fundus

9. The breasts contain these glands, which produce milk to nourish an infant:
   (A) Endometrial glands
   (B) Lactational glands
   (C) Sustenance glands
   (D) Mammary glands

10. This occurs when male and female gametes unite:
    (A) Menstruation
    (B) Fertilization
    (C) Lactation
    (D) Implantation

Name: ______________________

11. The X and Y sex chromosomes determine the baby's
    (A) Eye color
    (B) Height in adulthood
    (C) Sex
    (D) Athletic ability

12. A blastocyst releases this hormone, which signals the body to maintain and build up the uterine lining:
    (A) Estrogen
    (B) Progesterone
    (C) Human growth hormone
    (D) Human chorionic gonadotropin

13. This membrane surrounds a fetus and contains fluid that protects and supports it:
    (A) The placenta
    (B) The umbilical cord
    (C) The amniotic sac
    (D) The endometrium

True or False

14. ____ The uppermost section of the uterus is called the *cervix*.

15. ____ Fluid excreted from the bulbourethral glands removes acidity from the urethra, creating a better environment for semen.

16. ____ The labia and external vaginal opening are called the *vulva*.

17. ____ The male and female gametes each contribute 46 chromosomes.

18. ____ A fertilized egg is called a fetus.

2. Discuss lifespan changes to the reproductive system

Lifespan Changes for Females

Short Answer

1. List three secondary sex characteristics in females.

____

____

____

2. What is true of the ovaries at birth?

____

____

____

3. List three changes a woman may experience during perimenopause.

____

____

____

____

4. When does menopause occur?

____

____

____

____

5. Why may women be at risk for osteoporosis as they age?

____

____

____

____

Lifespan Changes for Males

Fill in the Blank

6. The testes form in the abdominal cavity and ______________ into the scrotum late in pregnancy or ______________ after birth.

7. During puberty, ______________ production begins, stimulated by follicle-stimulating hormone and luteinizing hormone.

8. Secondary sex characteristics include growth of ____________ hair, ______________ of the voice, and development of ______________ mass.

9. The amount of sperm produced ______________ with age.

10. As a man ages, the ______________ gland enlarges, which can interfere with ______________.

3. Discuss pregnancy, childbirth, and common disorders of pregnancy

Matching

Use each letter only once.

1. ____ Prenatal care
2. ____ Obstetrician/gynecologist
3. ____ Certified nurse-midwife
4. ____ First trimester
5. ____ Second trimester
6. ____ Third trimester
7. ____ Estimated due date

(A) From 29 to 40 weeks gestation

(B) The menstrual period stops and nausea and fatigue are common.

(C) Care of women during pregnancy

(D) When a pregnancy will be full-term

(E) A doctor who specializes in women's health care, including prenatal care and childbirth

(F) A nurse with graduate-level training in gynecological and prenatal care

(G) Fatigue and nausea are likely to improve.

Short Answer

Place a check mark (✓) beside items below that may be part of a routine prenatal examination.

8. ____ Nuchal translucency test
9. ____ Measuring fundal height
10. ____ Doppler of fetal heartbeat
11. ____ Chorionic villus sampling
12. ____ Measuring vital signs and weight
13. ____ Ultrasound
14. ____ Amniocentesis
15. ____ Checking fetal position starting at 36 weeks

Short Answer

For each of the following patients, calculate the estimated due date (EDD) and note the trimester of the pregnancy. Show how you find the EDD.

16. It is July 1, 2025. The first day of Jana's last menstrual period was October 6, 2024.

EDD calculation: ______________________

____

____

Trimester: ______________________

17. It is June 8, 2023. The first day of Blanca's last menstrual period was April 15, 2023.

EDD calculation: ______________________

____

____

Trimester: ______________________

18. It is May 30, 2024. The first day of Aisha's last menstrual period was February 13, 2024.

EDD calculation: ______________________

____

____

Trimester: ______________________

True or False

19. ____ Delivery, or childbirth, normally occurs between 37 and 42 weeks of pregnancy.
20. ____ A pregnant patient should go to the hospital for delivery as soon as contractions start.
21. ____ A first birth typically takes 6–12 hours of labor.
22. ____ The afterbirth includes the placenta and fetal membranes.
23. ____ An umbilical cord stump should be kept moistened and covered.
24. ____ An Apgar score is based on assessing a newborn in 10 categories.

Name: ______________________________

25. ____ A pediatrician or neonatologist cares for newborn infants.

26. ____ Postpartum depression is to be expected and resolves on its own.

27. ____ During the first year of life infants receive all nourishment from breast milk or formula.

28. ____ Neonates normally consume 1–2 ounces of formula every 2–3 hours.

Pregnancy Disorders

Matching

Use each letter only once.

29. ____ Anemia

30. ____ Gestational diabetes

31. ____ *Hyperemesis gravidarum*

32. ____ Placenta previa

33. ____ Placental abruption

34. ____ Preeclampsia

35. ____ Miscarriage

36. ____ Stillbirth

(A) Development of high blood sugar during pregnancy

(B) Implantation of the placenta low in the uterus, partially or completely covering the cervical outlet

(C) The death of a mature fetus before or during delivery

(D) Occurs due to extra nutrient demands of the growing fetus and the additional blood supply needed during pregnancy

(E) The death of an embryo or fetus in pregnancy, before it is able to survive outside the womb

(F) The sudden complete or partial separation of the placenta from the uterine wall

(G) Excessive nausea and vomiting, which usually occurs during the first trimester

(H) The sudden development of hypertension in pregnancy

4. List common chronic and acute conditions of the reproductive system

Conditions of the Male Reproductive System

Multiple Choice

1. Which of the following is true of prostate cancer?
   (A) It is rare.
   (B) Risk increases with age.
   (C) It is more common in younger men.
   (D) It usually grows aggressively and is difficult to treat.

2. In benign prostatic hyperplasia (BPH), prostate enlargement can lead to problems with this function:
   (A) Bowel elimination
   (B) Removing toxins from the blood
   (C) Maintaining fluid balance
   (D) Urination

3. About 10% of male infants are born with this condition:
   (A) Testicular cancer
   (B) Hydrocele
   (C) Benign prostatic hyperplasia
   (D) Pelvic inflammatory disease

4. What are the most common causes of erectile dysfunction?
   (A) Physical causes such as heart disease and high blood pressure
   (B) Abnormalities in the structure of the penis
   (C) Psychological factors such as stress
   (D) Lifestyle factors such as tobacco and alcohol use

5. What age group is most likely to be affected by testicular cancer?
   (A) Infants
   (B) Young adults
   (C) Adults in middle age
   (D) Elderly adults

Conditions of the Female Reproductive System

Short Answer

6. What types of microorganisms may cause vaginitis?

____

____

____

7. What is the most common cause of pelvic inflammatory disease?

____

____

8. List three of the conditions for which a woman has a higher risk after menopause.

____

____

____

____

9. Treatments for this condition include oral contraceptives, surgery, and (in severe cases) hysterectomy.

____

10. What is the best tool for early detection of breast cancer?

____

11. What is one way for a woman to reduce her risk of cervical cancer?

____

____

12. This form of cancer is more common in women after menopause and its signs and symptoms include abdominal pain, vaginal bleeding, and/or vaginal discharge.

____

Sexually Transmitted Infections

True or False

13. ____ Gonorrhea is easier to detect in men than in women.
14. ____ Genital herpes can be cured with antibiotics.
15. ____ Condoms can reduce the risk of transmission of some sexually transmitted infections.
16. ____ Gonorrhea can cause sterility.
17. ____ Symptoms of chlamydia include yellow or white discharge from the penis or vagina and a burning sensation during urination.
18. ____ Syphilis is a bacterial infection.
19. ____ Most women infected with gonorrhea show many early symptoms.
20. ____ Genital HPV infection is rare.
21. ____ Sexually transmitted infections can be transmitted through contact of the mouth with the genitals of an infected person.
22. ____ Genital HPV infection can be cured with a strong antibiotic.
23. ____ There is a vaccine available for HPV.

5. Describe examinations and procedures related to the reproductive system

Examination of the Male Reproductive System

Short Answer

Place a check mark (✓) beside items below that may be part of a routine examination of the male reproductive system.

1. ____ Testicular exam
2. ____ Assessment for an inguinal hernia
3. ____ Breast exam
4. ____ Digital rectal examination to palpate the prostate gland

5. ____ Pelvic exam

6. ____ Medical, social, and family history

Examination of the Female Reproductive System

Fill in the Blank

7. If a provider performs a clinical breast exam, each breast is palpated to check for ____________ or ____________.

8. A pelvic exam includes ______________ inspection of the vulva, vagina, and ____________.

9. A patient is in ______________ position for a pelvic exam.

10. During a pelvic exam, the provider examines the ____________ and ______________ by palpation.

11. A(n) ________ test is a test used to detect abnormal cells on the cervix.

12. Co-testing means testing cervical cells for both ________ changes and ________.

Multiple Choice

13. The following items are needed during a Pap test:
    (A) Cervical brush, microscope slides, and fixative
    (B) X-ray machine, sticky tabs to mark moles, and patient gown
    (C) Specimen cup, reagent strip, and interpretation key
    (D) Electrodes, wires, and adhesive gel

14. During a Pap test the MA may be responsible for
    (A) Applying fixative to microscope slides
    (B) Inserting the speculum
    (C) Using a brush to remove cervical cells
    (D) Using a microscope to examine cervical cells

15. Which of the following women may need to start having mammograms earlier than 45 years of age?
    (A) A woman who has never given birth
    (B) A woman who has given birth to more than two children
    (C) A woman with BRCA gene mutations
    (D) A woman with no family history of breast cancer

16. What is the name of the noninvasive instrument that allows the provider to have a magnified view of the cervix?
    (A) A speculum
    (B) A cervical brush
    (C) An intrauterine device
    (D) A colposcope

Contraceptive Counseling

Matching

Each letter may be used more than once.

17. ____ Oral contraceptives

18. ____ Natural family planning

19. ____ Tubal ligation

20. ____ Injected contraceptives

21. ____ Diaphragms

22. ____ *Coitus interruptus* (withdrawal, pull-out method)

23. ____ Implanted contraceptives

24. ____ Spermicides

25. ____ Condoms

26. ____ Vasectomy

27. ____ Cervical caps

28. ____ Transdermal contraceptives

29. ____ Emergency contraceptives

30. ____ Vaginal ring

31. ____ Intrauterine device

(A) Always involves the use of hormones

(B) More effective when used with a spermicide

(C) Can prevent the transmission of STIs

(D) Must be used within five days of intercourse

(E) Not as effective as other forms of birth control

(F) Surgical procedure performed on a male

(G) May be inserted in the vagina or added to barrier contraceptives

(H) Some types contain hormones and some do not

6. Discuss patient education related to the reproductive system

Scenarios

1. Marjorie's mother was diagnosed with breast cancer at age 50. Marjorie is only 22 but she wants to know how to perform breast self-examination. Her gynecologist asks MA Jessica to review guidelines for breast self-exam with her. How should Jessica instruct Marjorie?

2. Santiago's doctor sees that he has a family history of testicular cancer and asks her MA, Gideon, to provide education in testicular self-examination. What should Gideon tell Santiago to do?

3. Elizabeth is 19 years old and tells her gynecologist that she and her boyfriend are planning to become sexually active. Her gynecologist prescribes oral contraceptives and asks Jessica to review how to take the oral contraceptives. What should Jessica make sure Elizabeth understands?

Name: ______________________________

4. Because oral contraceptives do not protect against STIs, Elizabeth's gynecologist also asks Jessica to review information about STI prevention. What should Jessica tell Elizabeth?

____

____

____

____

____

____

____

____

____

____

____

____

23

The Immune and Lymphatic Systems and Related Care

1. Describe the structure and function of the immune and lymphatic systems

Short Answer

1. What is the difference between nonspecific immunity and specific immunity?

2. List three defenses that are part of the body's nonspecific immune response.

3. Describe the two types of lymphocytes.

4. What are two ways a person can gain active immunity to a disease?

5. What are two ways a person can gain passive immunity?

Multiple Choice

6. How is lymph fluid circulated?
   (A) It is pumped out by the heart.
   (B) The thymus gland acts as a pump.
   (C) Muscle activity, massage, and breathing circulate it.
   (D) The bone marrow acts as a pump.

7. Which of the following is one of the functions of the spleen?
   (A) Creating T cells
   (B) Training T cells to recognize foreign antigens
   (C) Storing blood cells
   (D) Absorbing fats and fat-soluble nutrients

8. Where are all red blood cells, all platelets, and many white blood cells produced?
   (A) In the lymph nodes
   (B) In the bone marrow
   (C) In the thymus
   (D) In the appendix

Name: ________________________

9. Which of these lists only includes structures that are part of the lymphatic system?
   (A) Lymph nodes, lymph vessels, tonsils, Peyer's patches, appendix, spleen
   (B) Lymph nodes, lymph vessels, appendix, gallbladder, lacteals, spleen
   (C) Bone marrow, appendix, tonsils, bronchi, Peyer's patches, lymph nodes
   (D) Lacteals, heart, spleen, tonsils, lymph nodes, lymph vessels

2. Discuss lifespan changes to the immune and lymphatic systems

Fill in the Blank

1. At birth, a newborn infant has a(n) ________________ amount of immunity to disease from transfer of the mother's ________________.
2. This immunity ________________ over the first few months of life.
3. The thymus gland is most active in ______________ and ________________.
4. As a person ages, the response to vaccines ________________.
5. An older person may be less able to contract a(n) ____________ to fight infection.
6. It is normal for the immune system to ________________ with age, increasing the risk of all types of ________________.

3. List common chronic and acute conditions of the immune and lymphatic systems

Short Answer

1. Describe three medical specialties associated with the immune and lymphatic systems.

____

____

____

____

____

____

____

2. List three possible subspecialities of oncology.

____

____

____

____

Allergies

True or False

3. ____ Allergies can be mild or life-threatening.
4. ____ Allergic reactions happen when a toxic substance triggers an immune response.
5. ____ Anaphylaxis is a severe reaction to an allergen and must be treated immediately.
6. ____ Common allergens include oatmeal, apples, and mosquito bites.

Bacterial and Viral Infections

Multiple Choice

7. As appendicitis worsens, where does the pain move?
   (A) Toward the center of the chest
   (B) Toward the right lower quadrant of the abdomen
   (C) Toward the left lower quadrant of the abdomen
   (D) Toward the stomach
8. Appendicitis is treated with surgery to remove the appendix because
   (A) It is too painful to endure
   (B) The appendix has no purpose in the body
   (C) The appendix may rupture and spread the infection throughout the abdomen
   (D) It is caused by a virus and so cannot be treated with antibiotics

9. Epstein-Barr virus may cause the bone marrow to
   (A) Create too many white blood cells
   (B) Stop creating white blood cells
   (C) Create too many red blood cells
   (D) Atrophy

10. Mononucleosis is spread easily through contact with an infected person's
   (A) Saliva
   (B) Sweat
   (C) Hands
   (D) Blood

Lymphedema/Autoimmune Illnesses

Fill in the Blank

11. Lymphedema often occurs after _______________ surgery.

12. Lymphedema is the abnormal buildup of ______________________________ in the body's tissues.

13. Lymph fluid is drained from the extremities through exercise, special massage therapy called ______________________________ ______________________, and the use of _______________ devices.

14. Blood pressure measurement and ______________________ should not be performed in a limb affected by lymphedema.

15. Psoriasis, rheumatoid arthritis, myasthenia gravis, and multiple sclerosis are all _______________ conditions.

16. The most common form of lupus is systemic lupus ______________________________.

17. SLE can cause symptoms in many parts of the body, but the _____________, kidneys, and ___________ are most often affected.

18. Drugs that are typically used to prevent or treat _______________ change the immune system in a way that can relieve lupus symptoms.

Acquired Immunodeficiency Syndrome (AIDS)

True or False

19. ____ HIV and AIDS are the same illness.

20. ____ HIV can only be transmitted through sexual contact.

21. ____ The first stage of HIV infection involves symptoms similar to flu.

22. ____ The diagnosis of AIDS is made when a person first begins to have symptoms of illness.

23. ____ AIDS dementia complex results from damage to the central nervous system.

24. ____ Opportunistic infections such as pneumonia can cause death in people with AIDS.

25. ____ A vaccine to prevent HIV and AIDS is widely available.

26. ____ An effective treatment called antiretroviral therapy involves taking combinations of medications every day.

27. ____ Pre-exposure prophylaxis is a way to protect patients with AIDS from opportunistic infections.

28. ____ It can take as long as 3–6 months for HIV to be detected by testing.

29. ____ HIV testing can be performed without a person's consent.

30. ____ A healthcare worker with HIV or AIDS may be fired to prevent transmission of the disease.

Cancer

Multiple Choice

31. How does cancer spread through the body in lymphoma?
   (A) Via the bone marrow
   (B) Via the lymph nodes
   (C) Via the bloodstream
   (D) Via the thymus

32. Multiple myeloma reduces room for
    (A) Mature B cells
    (B) Red blood cells
    (C) Lymph fluid
    (D) Food in the digestive system

33. What is true of cancer treatment after cancer has metastasized?
    (A) It is easier.
    (B) It is no longer possible.
    (C) It is more difficult.
    (D) Only surgery is possible.

34. Cancer is categorized by
    (A) Stage and grade
    (B) Level and strength
    (C) Location and size
    (D) Color and thickness

35. The key treatment for malignant tumors of the skin, breast, bladder, colon, rectum, stomach, and muscle is
    (A) Surgery
    (B) Homeopathic pills
    (C) Radiation
    (D) Hormone therapy

36. Nausea, vomiting, diarrhea, hair loss, and decreased resistance to infection are all side effects of which treatment?
    (A) Surgery
    (B) Chemotherapy
    (C) Cold applications
    (D) Herbal remedies

37. This treatment method uses medications intravenously to destroy cancer cells and limit the rate of cell growth:
    (A) Surgery
    (B) Chemotherapy
    (C) Radiation
    (D) Herbal remedies

38. This treatment method involves removing as much of the tumor as possible to prevent cancer from spreading:
    (A) Surgery
    (B) Chemotherapy
    (C) Radiation
    (D) Hormone therapy

39. This treatment method kills normal and abnormal cells in a limited area, sometimes causing skin to become sore, irritated, or burned:
    (A) Surgery
    (B) Chemotherapy
    (C) Radiation
    (D) Immunotherapy

4. Describe examinations and procedures related to the immune and lymphatic systems

Short Answer

1. What structures are palpated during examination of the lymphatic system and where are they located?

____

____

____

2. Why are blood tests and diagnostic imaging often used to assess the lymphatic system?

____

____

____

____

3. List three forms of diagnostic imaging that may be used.

____

____

____

4. Describe three methods of allergy testing.

____

____

____

____

____

5. What are two ways to label allergens during allergy testing?

____

____

____

____

____

____

6. What is a control solution and how is it used in allergy testing?

____

____

____

____

____

____

____

____

____

____

7. How many needles or lancets are needed for allergy testing?

____

____

____

____

____

True or False

8. ____ The goal of allergy injections is to increase the patient's immune response to the allergens.

9. ____ Because of the risk of an anaphylactic reaction, the MA should monitor patients carefully for 20–30 minutes after allergy injections.

10. ____ An antibody titer is a blood test to measure a person's immunity to a specific disease.

11. ____ Patients who are receiving cancer treatment may receive regular subcutaneous injections to boost the body's production of insulin.

12. ____ An MA's main role in assisting with a biopsy is to study the tissues the provider removes.

13. ____ Tests that may be ordered to detect abnormal tissue when cancer is suspected include CT scans, MRIs, and PET scans.

14. ____ Part of an MA's role in caring for patients with cancer is to have a list of resources available for such things as wigs and compression sleeves.

5. Discuss patient education related to the immune and lymphatic systems

Crossword

Across

4. Patients must be taught that blood should never be drawn on the same side where this type of operation was done.
5. Vitamin E is found in this type of tree nut.
7. Sun exposure and fortified dairy products are sources.

Name: ______________________________

Down

1. This type of activity is vital to lymph circulation.
2. Keeping up-to-date with these ensures protection against many illnesses.
3. This is one of the minerals needed for the production of blood cells.
6. Wearing this during flu season or a COVID-19 surge can protect against infection.

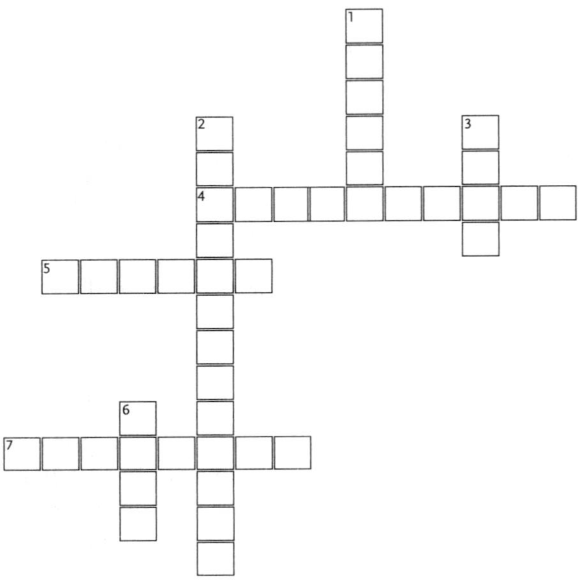

24

Phlebotomy and Common Blood Tests

1. Discuss venipuncture and capillary puncture and identify common blood tests

Matching

Use each letter only once.

1. _____ Dermal puncture
2. _____ Blood cultures
3. _____ Venipuncture
4. _____ Test panel
5. _____ Point-of-care tests
6. _____ Blood smear
7. _____ Iatrogenic anemia

(A) A way to test for bacterial or fungal infections

(B) Allows blood cells to be viewed under a microscope

(C) Another term for *capillary puncture*, or puncturing the skin to collect a blood specimen

(D) A group of blood tests with related analytes or that relate to a specific condition or organ

(E) A condition caused by removing too much blood from a patient

(F) The puncture of a vein; done to draw a blood specimen

(G) Tests performed at the patient's side; glucose and blood clotting times are often tested this way

Short Answer

Place a check mark (✓) beside the descriptions of patients who may need to have blood specimens taken by capillary puncture rather than venipuncture.

8. _____ Patients with burned or heavily scarred arms
9. _____ Patients who are between the ages of 2 and 12
10. _____ Patients who are dehydrated
11. _____ Patients whose veins are very fragile or damaged
12. _____ Patients whose veins are difficult to see
13. _____ Patients whose veins must be used only for treatments such as chemotherapy
14. _____ Patients who have bruises on their hands

2. Describe the importance of avoiding errors before and during specimen collection

Multiple Choice

1. Which of the following is true of a specimen that is not collected properly?
   (A) It may provide inaccurate test results.
   (B) It is not a problem as long as the right amount is collected.
   (C) It is not a problem as long as it is collected in the correct tube.
   (D) It is not a problem as long as the MA tells the lab that an error occurred.

2. What is the term for errors that occur with a specimen before it is tested?
   (A) Pretest problems
   (B) Collection mistakes
   (C) Venipuncture errors
   (D) Preanalytical errors
3. What must be done before a specimen is drawn?
   (A) The MA must label all specimen tubes.
   (B) The MA should assure the patient that everything will be fine.
   (C) The MA should properly identify the patient using two unique identifiers.
   (D) The MA should ask the patient to confirm their name.
4. This common patient requirement before a blood draw involves not eating or drinking anything other than water for 8–12 hours:
   (A) Abstaining
   (B) Fasting
   (C) Thickened liquids only
   (D) NPO
5. Which of these is considered an error?
   (A) Mixing a specimen with the chemical additive in a tube
   (B) Using a butterfly needle on a geriatric patient
   (C) Not filling multiple collection tubes in the correct order
   (D) Asking the patient if he has had anything to eat

3. Identify equipment used to collect blood specimens

True or False

1. ____ A multisample needle allows an MA to collect more than 1 tube of blood while puncturing the patient's vein only once.
2. ____ MAs must pump air out of most collection tubes before using them.
3. ____ After drawing blood, the MA must remove the needle from the tube holder and discard it in the sharps receptacle.
4. ____ The hollow space inside a needle is called a bevel.
5. ____ The higher the gauge number of a needle, the thinner the needle.
6. ____ A winged collection set and a butterfly assembly are the same thing.
7. ____ Specimens for blood cultures must never be collected using a butterfly assembly.
8. ____ Evacuated tube systems create pressure on a patient's veins.
9. ____ A syringe may be used when collecting blood from a patient with thin or fragile veins.
10. ____ Blood collected in a syringe is sent to the lab in the syringe barrel.

Matching

Use each letter only once.

11. ____ Gloves
12. ____ Antiseptic solution
13. ____ Tourniquet
14. ____ Gauze
15. ____ Bandage
16. ____ Warming pack
17. ____ Venoscope
18. ____ Microcollection tubes
19. ____ Lancet
20. ____ Test strips

(A) Applying pressure on this after venipuncture helps stop the flow of blood.

(B) An electronic device that may be used to aid in vein location

(C) Term for tubes used to collect capillary specimens

(D) Placed over the gauze after bleeding has stopped

(E) Should not have holes; should not be torn to palpate the patient's veins

(F) May be required for glucose or PT/INR testing

(G) The most commonly used is 70% isopropyl alcohol.

(H) Devices with a retractable needle or blade; used to start blood flow for capillary specimens

(I) Makes it easier to find a patient's veins

(J) Can make veins easier to find and improve blood flow for capillary puncture

4. Identify additives to blood specimens and list the order in which collection tubes must be filled (order of draw)

Fill in the Blank

1. Tube stoppers are color coded based on the type of ________________ inside.
2. ________________ is the liquid that is left after blood has clotted in a collection tube.
3. Some tubes include clot ____________________ to make specimens clot faster.
4. When a specimen with anticoagulants is spun in a centrifuge, it divides into _____________ and solid components.
5. In addition to chemical additives that act on the blood, tubes may contain a(n) _______________ gel that forms a barrier between the solids and liquids after centrifugation.
6. Right after a blood draw, a specimen with an additive must be gently turned upside down and then brought _______________ several times. This motion is called a(n) __________________.
7. Chemical additives can __________________ from one tube to the next when the tubes are changed.
8. Using the correct order of draw prevents clot activators, for example, from getting into a tube with a(n) ____________________________.

Short Answer

9. List the CLSI order of draw for venipuncture.

____
____
____
____
____
____
____
____
____
____
____
____

10. An MA needs to draw a lavender tube, a light blue tube, and a green tube. In what order should they be drawn?

____
____

11. A patient needs a blood culture and also needs a light blue tube drawn. What will the MA draw first?

____
____

12. Why is order of draw different for capillary collections?

____
____
____
____
____
____
____

13. What is the order of draw for capillary collections?

____

____

____

____

____

5. Understand the importance of safety during the collection of blood specimens

Short Answer

1. When must an MA wear gloves during a blood draw?

____

____

2. Where should the sharps container be while an MA is drawing blood?

____

____

3. When is a sharps container considered to be full?

____

____

4. What can an MA do to be ready for unexpected challenges before they arise?

____

____

____

____

____

____

6. Identify appropriate sites for venipuncture and capillary puncture

Multiple Choice

1. Where on the body is venipuncture most often done?
   (A) On the dorsal aspect of the hand
   (B) On the wrist
   (C) In the antecubital fossa
   (D) On the lateral plantar surface of the foot

2. Which of the following is a reason the median cubital vein is the first choice for venipuncture?
   (A) It always produces good blood flow.
   (B) It is never painful to puncture.
   (C) It is easy to reach.
   (D) It is well anchored and not close to arteries or nerves.

3. Which vein should be the last choice for venipuncture?
   (A) The cephalic vein
   (B) The basilic vein
   (C) The lateral antebrachial vein
   (D) The medial antebrachial vein

4. What is the best way to find a good vein for venipuncture?
   (A) By palpation
   (B) By sight
   (C) By asking the patient which vein is best
   (D) By probing with the needle

5. How should a healthy vein feel?
   (A) Ropy and dense
   (B) Hard and bumpy
   (C) Soft and movable
   (D) Springy and uniform

6. If a patient's veins are located relatively deep under the skin, the MA should
   (A) Insert the needle at a lower angle
   (B) Insert the needle at a higher angle
   (C) Use a longer needle
   (D) Use a shorter needle

7. Why should a patient not pump their fist while the MA looks for a vein?
   (A) It will make the puncture uncomfortable.
   (B) Pumping the fist with a tourniquet in place can cause the vein to pop.
   (C) It can cause hemoconcentration and/or hemolysis.
   (D) It can cause the arm to move, which makes it harder to find the vein.

8. When is it appropriate to use a vein in the hand for venipuncture?
   (A) When a vein in the inner elbow cannot be found or cannot be used
   (B) Any time the MA is using a butterfly needle
   (C) Any time a specimen is being drawn for blood culture
   (D) When the patient is a young child

Scenarios

9. Ali is assigned to perform capillary puncture on Joseph, an adult patient. Joseph is a professional violinist and the fingers of his left hand are calloused. He is right-handed. Ali does not want to use the dominant hand. He decides to puncture the very tip of Joseph's ring finger on his left hand because the skin is smoother there. Was this a good decision? Why or why not?

____
____
____
____
____
____
____
____
____

10. Rowan is a newborn infant. Martina is an MA at a birth center and is assigned to perform capillary puncture for newborn screening. She punctures Rowan's right heel, roughly in line with her smallest toe. Was this a good decision? Why or why not?

____
____
____
____
____
____
____
____
____
____

11. Marilu had a double mastectomy five years ago. MA Johanna is assigned by a *locum tenens* provider who does not know Marilu's history to draw blood for a complete blood count using a lavender tube (venipuncture). Marilu tells her that she's had finger sticks before with no problem. Johanna performs capillary puncture and collects the specimen in a lavender microcollection tube. Was this a good decision? Why or why not?

____
____
____
____
____
____
____
____

Name: ______________________

12. Dorothy is a patient who comes in regularly for PT/INR testing. On a hot summer day, MA Austen can see that Dorothy has very swollen hands and feet. Austen is concerned that edema will interfere with the test results. She asks Dorothy to please wait a moment while she speaks to the provider. Was this a good decision? Why or why not?

____

____

____

____

____

____

____

____

____

____

7. Describe site preparation and proper needle/lancet placement

True or False

1. ____ Current CLSI standards say that a venipuncture site must be cleaned in concentric circles.
2. ____ Blowing on a blood draw site after cleaning is an effective way to dry the antiseptic agent.
3. ____ Sites for blood culture specimen collection must be cleaned more thoroughly than sites for other tests.
4. ____ Povidone-iodine should not be used on patients with shellfish allergies.
5. ____ The angle of needle insertion for venipuncture should be higher than 30 degrees.
6. ____ Putting the needle straight through a vein is referred to as a *blown vein.*
7. ____ Probing blindly for a vein can cause pain and create a hematoma.
8. ____ If blood does not start to flow after puncturing the vein, the MA can gently adjust the needle slightly forward or slightly back.
9. ____ The tourniquet should remain on the patient's arm as long as it takes to successfully locate and access a patient's vein.
10. ____ An MA should only make one venipuncture attempt on a patient. If it fails, the MA should tell the provider.
11. ____ A blade-style lancet should be placed at a 90-degree angle (perpendicular) to a patient's fingerprint lines.
12. ____ The longer a capillary collection takes, the more likely the blood is to clump.

8. Describe procedures for routine venipuncture and capillary puncture

Fill in the Blank

1. Most venipuncture procedures are done in the ________________ area of the arm with a straight ______________ multisample needle and evacuated tubes.
2. Expired or damaged equipment must be properly ______________________.
3. A tourniquet cannot stay in place for more than ____________________________.
4. After the vein is punctured, the tourniquet is ________________________ as soon as blood flow begins.
5. For all types of blood draws, if the patient is a young child, the MA should request that the parent or guardian _______________ the child during the procedure.
6. Tell the patient that she may feel brief _____________ as the needle enters the skin.
7. In a(n) _______________, _______________ motion, insert the needle into the skin to puncture the selected vein.

8. Most citrate and serum tubes require ______________ inversions; most other tubes require ____________.

9. After venipuncture, bleeding may take as long as ________________ to stop for patients on anticoagulant medications.

10. When using a syringe transfer device, do not ______________ the syringe plunger as the blood transfers. The ______________ in the tube will draw blood in to the required level.

11. For infants under _______ months old and who weigh less than _____ pounds, the capillary puncture site is the medial or lateral plantar surface of either heel.

12. During capillary puncture collections, do not ______________ or ______________ the finger or heel.

13. Gently ____________ the collection tube while collecting a capillary specimen helps mix the specimen.

14. Always label specimens ______________________ the patient and after the collection is complete.

15. If a patient is feeling faint before a blood draw or reports a history of fainting, the correct position for the patient during the draw is reclined or ________________.

9. Identify guidelines for processing and transporting specimens

Matching

Use each letter only once.

1. ____ Centrifugation
2. ____ Aliquots
3. ____ Pipette
4. ____ Serum tubes
5. ____ Serum filter
6. ____ Heating block
7. ____ Ice slurry

(A) Mixture of crushed ice and water used to keep specimens cold

(B) Device inserted into a specimen tube to prevent the solid materials from mixing with the liquid portion

(C) Smaller amounts taken from a larger specimen for testing

(D) Rack designed to hold tubes upright at a specific temperature

(E) Spinning of samples to separate solid and liquid components

(F) Must be allowed to clot fully before centrifugation

(G) A narrow tube with a suction bulb; used to remove the liquid portion of a specimen

Multiple Choice

8. What does it mean to balance a centrifuge load?
   (A) To only centrifuge tubes with the same chemical additive
   (B) To only centrifuge tubes of the same size
   (C) To place tubes evenly within the centrifuge
   (D) To only centrifuge specimens one time

9. CLSI standards require centrifugation within __________ of collection, but some specimens may need to be centrifuged sooner.
   (A) 30 minutes
   (B) 1 hour
   (C) 2 hours
   (D) 1 day

10. Plasma or serum should be
    (A) Cloudy and milky
    (B) Tinted orange
    (C) Tinted deep yellow
    (D) Clear and straw-colored

11. When separating serum or plasma, how should an MA remove the stopper from a specimen?
    (A) Using a special tool, if available, or carefully by hand
    (B) With a standard bottle opener
    (C) By popping it off with the thumb
    (D) By gently knocking it against the counter

12. Which of the following is an acceptable way to protect light-sensitive specimens?
    (A) By completing the draw in a darkened room
    (B) By using an amber or foil-wrapped collection tube
    (C) By asking the patient to hold the tube in cupped hands to block light
    (D) By placing the tube in a centrifuge immediately after collection and closing the lid

13. A lipemic specimen is most likely in which of the following cases?
    (A) The patient has been fasting.
    (B) The patient is jaundiced.
    (C) The collection tube was shaken to mix, rather than being inverted gently.
    (D) The patient had a breakfast of bacon and eggs.

10. Describe guidelines for performing point-of-care tests on capillary blood

Short Answer

1. What does a PT/INR test measure?

____

____

____

____

2. Who can perform CLIA-waived tests?

____

____

3. What should an MA do if asked to perform a point-of-care test using a device she has never used before?

____

____

____

4. Manufacturer instructions may include doing this before using a testing device.

____

____

5. What should an MA do when a result falls in the critical value range for a test?

____

____

____

____

____

6. How should test strips or containers be discarded?

____

____

7. Who should discuss results of point-of-care testing with patients?

____

____

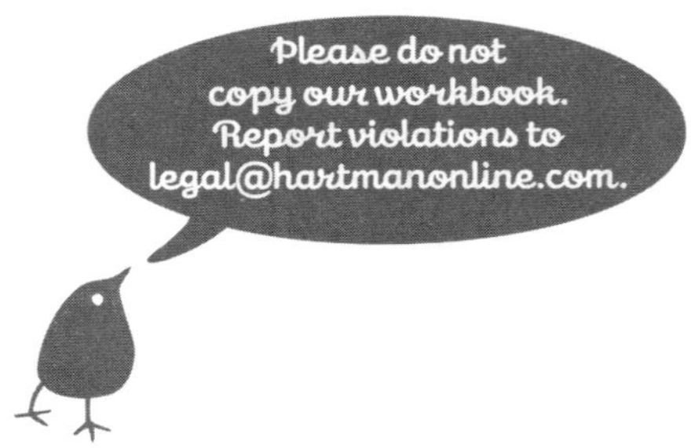

Name: ______________________________

25

Electrocardiograms (EKGs) and Related Tests

1. Describe the electrical activity of the heart and how it is recorded by EKG machines

Matching

Use each letter only once.

1. _____ Depolarization
2. _____ Repolarization
3. _____ Cardiac conduction
4. _____ SA node
5. _____ Electrodes
6. _____ Leads
7. _____ Mechanical activity
8. _____ Electrocardiogram (EKG)
9. _____ Echocardiogram

(A) Movement of electrical signals in the heart

(B) Pads that conduct electricity

(C) Change in electrical charge from positive back to negative

(D) Muscle contractions of the heart

(E) Primary pacemaker of the heart; sets timing of the heart's contractions

(F) Test that records the electrical activity of the heart

(G) Test that shows the mechanical activity of the heart

(H) Change in electrical charge from negative to positive

(I) "Views" of the heart's electrical activity recorded on an EKG

2. Understand EKG waveforms and identify normal features in an EKG

Crossword

Across

2. Upward and downward movements on an EKG tracing
4. The P wave shows depolarization of this part of the heart.
6. Normal sinus rhythm on an EKG can look __________ from person to person.
7. Several waves together

Down

1. The QRS complex shows this happening to the ventricles.
3. The isoelectric line on an EKG tracing is also called this.
5. Portion of an EKG tracing where the tracing goes back to the isoelectric line

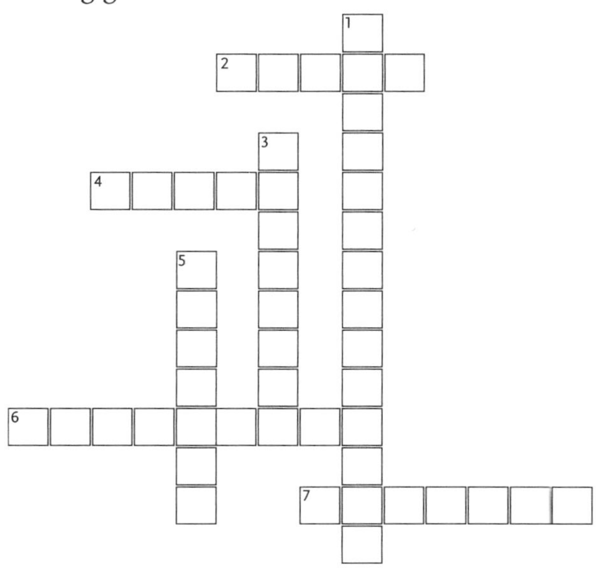

Name: ______________________________

3. Describe the types of EKG-based tests and how each is used

Scenarios

For each of the following scenarios, list the type of EKG testing most likely to be used.

1. Pat, age 72, has been having a fluttering sensation in her chest. She has also had periods of feeling lightheaded. An EKG at her doctor's office does not show any abnormalities, but the doctor would like to have information about her cardiac activity over a longer period.

____

2. Sean, age 58, is hospitalized overnight for observation after a minor heart attack.

____

3. Pablo, age 52, is an avid runner with a family history of heart disease. He reports to his cardiologist that he has recently experienced palpitations and shortness of breath, but only during exercise.

____

4. Sara, age 40, is at her PCP's office for a routine physical.

____

4. Describe EKG leads and electrode placement

Fill in the Blank

1. The limb leads are also called the ______________ leads.
2. Leads aVR, aVL, and aVF are called the ______________ limb leads.
3. Leads V1, V2, V3, V4, V5, and V6 are known together as the precordial leads, or ______________ leads.
4. The augmented limb leads and the precordial leads are not bipolar leads. They are ______________ leads.
5. One of the most common mistakes in electrocardiography is the ______________ of limb leads.
6. In 3-lead and 5-lead EKG applications the limb electrodes are placed on the ______________.
7. During a resting 12-lead EKG the limb electrodes may be placed on the ______________ or on the ______________.
8. A 12-lead EKG uses ______________ electrodes.

Labeling

For each electrode shown in the illustration, list the name of the electrode and describe its placement.

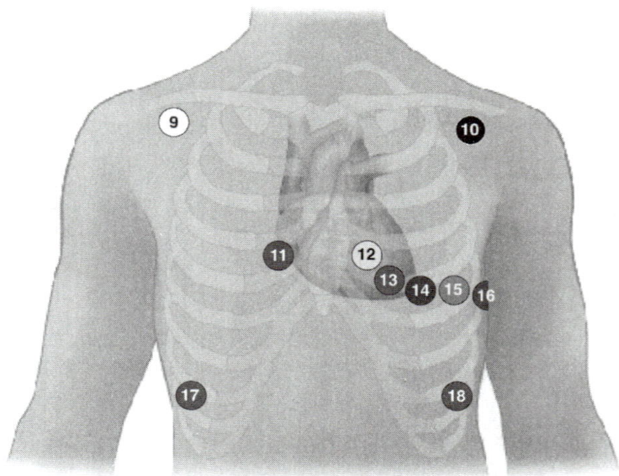

9. Electrode name: ______________________________

Placement: ______________________________

____

10. Electrode name: ______________________________

Placement: ______________________________

____

11. Electrode name: ______________________________

Placement: ______________________________

____

12. Electrode name: ______________________________

Placement: ______________________________

____

13. Electrode name: ____________________

Placement: ____________________

____

14. Electrode name: ____________________

Placement: ____________________

____

15. Electrode name: ____________________

Placement: ____________________

____

16. Electrode name: ____________________

Placement: ____________________

____

17. Electrode name: ____________________

Placement: ____________________

____

18. Electrode name: ____________________

Placement: ____________________

____

Multiple Choice

19. Which of the following is true for electrode placement on a patient with dextrocardia?
   (A) It is the same as standard electrode placement.
   (B) Chest electrodes are placed in a mirror image of standard electrode placement.
   (C) Electrodes V4, V5, and V6 are placed on the patient's back.
   (D) It is the same as standard electrode placement, but electrode V4 is moved to the right side of the chest.

20. On a patient with an above-knee amputation of the left leg, an MA places the LL electrode on the front of the left thigh. Where should the RL electrode be placed?
   (A) Immediately next to the LL electrode
   (B) On the lower right torso
   (C) Near the right ankle
   (D) On the front of the right thigh, mirroring the LL placement

21. In what situation might a provider request a posterior EKG?
   (A) The patient has a limb amputation.
   (B) The patient has scar tissue on the chest wall.
   (C) The provider suspects the patient has had a certain type of heart attack.
   (D) The patient prefers it to a standard EKG.

22. How are electrodes placed when doing an EKG on a 15-year-old patient?
   (A) In the standard locations
   (B) In the same positions as for a patient with dextrocardia
   (C) In the standard locations, but electrode V4 is moved to the right side of the chest
   (D) With electrodes V4, V5, and V6 on the patient's back

23. How should a woman in her seventh month of pregnancy be positioned for an EKG?
   (A) Supine position
   (B) Sims' position
   (C) Tilted slightly to the right
   (D) Tilted slightly to the left

5. Demonstrate the performance of the 12-lead EKG test

Short Answer

1. Where should an EKG machine be placed during testing?

____

____

____

2. What is the default paper speed on an EKG machine?

____

3. Why might a provider request that an EKG be run at a faster paper speed?

____

____

____

____

____

4. What does *gain* measure?

____

____

____

5. At default speed and default gain, what should the measurements of an EKG calibration mark be?

____

____

6. What steps might an MA need to take to help electrodes stick to the patient's skin?

____

____

____

7. What should the MA report to the provider immediately regarding an EKG?

____

____

____

8. An MA should take care not to do this when removing lead wires.

____

____

6. Demonstrate the performance of a stress test

Fill in the Blank

1. Stress tests may be used as a(n) ______________________ tool for patients 35 years of age and older, especially those with a(n) ______________________ of heart disease.
2. Exercise on a(n) ______________________ or stationary bicycle is the most common way of raising a patient's heart rate for a stress test.
3. Patients scheduled for a stress test should avoid ______________________ for 24 hours before the exam. This means avoiding ______________________, tea, some soft drinks, chocolate, and certain ______________________ medications.
4. Some medications may need to be ______________________ temporarily.
5. The patient should wear ______________________, loose clothing, and rubber-soled or ______________ shoes.
6. The stress test procedure lasts ______________ hour(s).

Short Answer

7. Pablo is 52 years old. What heart rate must he reach in order for his stress test to be valid? Show how you find the rate. Round to the nearest whole number as needed.

____

____

____

____

____

8. Jenny is 48 years old. What heart rate must she reach in order for her stress test to be valid? Show how you find the rate. Round to the nearest whole number as needed.

____

____

____

____

____

9. List five signs/symptoms that should cause a stress test to be stopped immediately.

____

____

____

____

____

____

____

____

7. Discuss Holter and other ambulatory monitoring

Multiple Choice

1. Why is it especially important to place electrodes securely for ambulatory monitoring?
   (A) Because patients often try to pull them off
   (B) Because patients will be wearing the monitor for 24 hours or more and will continue regular activities
   (C) Because electrodes designed for ambulatory monitoring have weaker adhesive
   (D) Because patients will be showering with the electrodes in place

2. How many electrodes are used for most forms of ambulatory monitoring?
   (A) 3
   (B) 5
   (C) 10
   (D) 12

3. What may be sent with the patient, along with instructions for replacement if needed?
   (A) Extra batteries
   (B) Extra lead wires
   (C) Extra paper to record the tracing
   (D) An extra monitoring unit

4. What basic medical supply can an MA use to create stress loops if the facility's electrodes do not have a clip or slot?
   (A) Gauze
   (B) A 70% isopropyl alcohol prep pad
   (C) Tape
   (D) Self-adhering bandage wrap

Short Answer

Place a check mark (✓) beside common patient education points for Holter monitoring.

5. ____ You may shower and swim with the Holter monitor in place.

6. ____ Call the provider's office if the electrodes become loose or fall off.

7. ____ Continue your normal activities.

8. ____ Keep an activity or symptom diary. Press the event button on the monitor for any concerning symptom.

9. ____ Call 911 for any palpitations or "skipped" heartbeats.

10. ____ Return all equipment as directed when the test is complete.

8. Demonstrate solutions to different types of EKG artifact

Matching

Match each type of artifact with a possible cause and solution. Write two letters on the answer blank for each artifact: one for a cause and one for a solution. Use each letter only once.

1. __________ Somatic tremor

2. __________ Wandering baseline

3. __________ Electrical interference

4. __________ Broken recording

Causes:

(A) The EKG machine is plugged in close to another electrical device.

(B) The patient applied lotion to her skin just before coming in for the EKG.

(C) The patient is cold and is shivering.

(D) The lead wires are frayed.

Solutions:

(E) Clean the skin with soap and water, then dry thoroughly.

(F) Offer the patient a blanket; ask him to put his hands under his buttocks.

(G) Replace frayed wires.

(H) Turn off the other device and/or plug the EKG machine into a different outlet.

Multiple Choice

5. On an EKG tracing, somatic tremor artifact causes
   (A) A fine, choppy distortion
   (B) A baseline that goes up and down across the tracing
   (C) A heavy, blurring interference
   (D) The stylus to go from side to side searching for a signal

6. When the baseline goes up and down across an EKG tracing, the MA should first check
   (A) That the electrodes are placed securely
   (B) That the patient is not cold or trembling
   (C) That no other appliances are plugged in near the EKG machine
   (D) That wires are not frayed

9. Identify normal and abnormal heart rhythms

True or False

1. ____ Heart rhythm and heart rate are the same thing.

2. ____ A normal heart rhythm has a clear P wave that is the same from beat to beat.

3. ____ Dysrhythmias may be too fast, too slow, or start in an area of the heart other than the SA node.

4. ____ Atrial rhythms have wide QRS complexes.

5. ____ Heart block rhythms may have long spaces between the P wave and the R wave.

6. ____ Pacemakers do not change the appearance of an EKG.

7. ____ An elevated ST segment may indicate a cardiac emergency, but a depressed ST segment is normal.

8. ____ An MA is not responsible for identifying heart rhythms, but should know what a normal EKG looks like.

Short Answer

Circle the EKG tracings below that show an ***abnormal*** *heart rhythm.*

9.

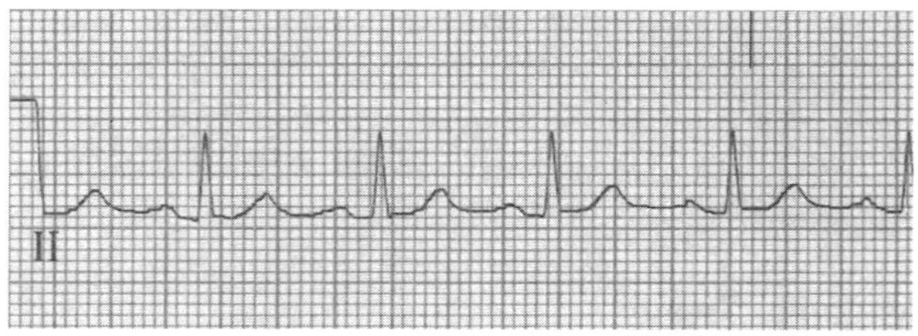

10.

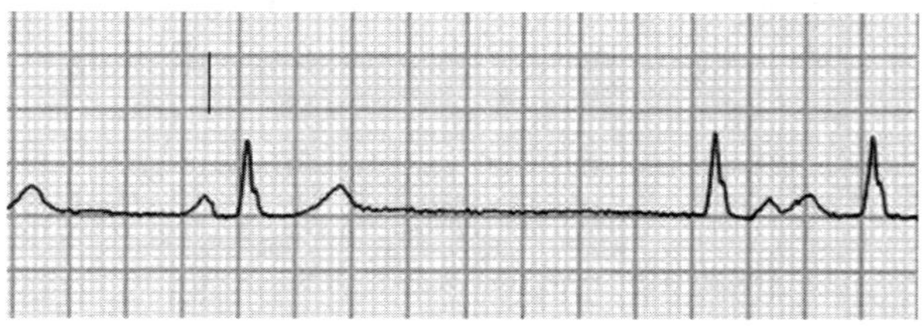

11.

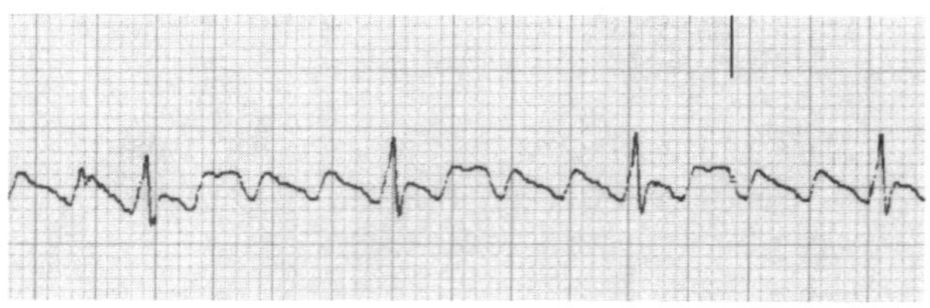

12.

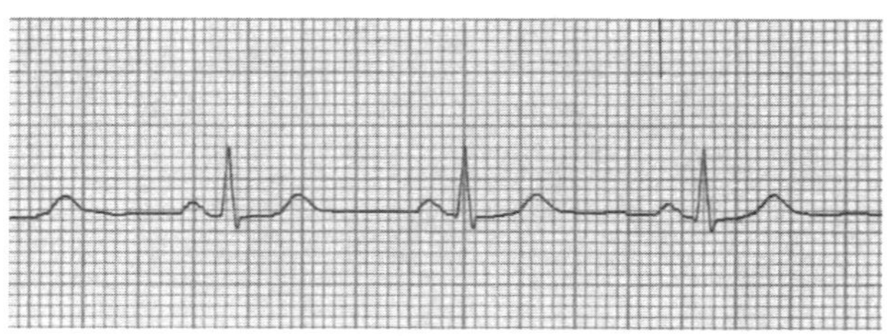

13.

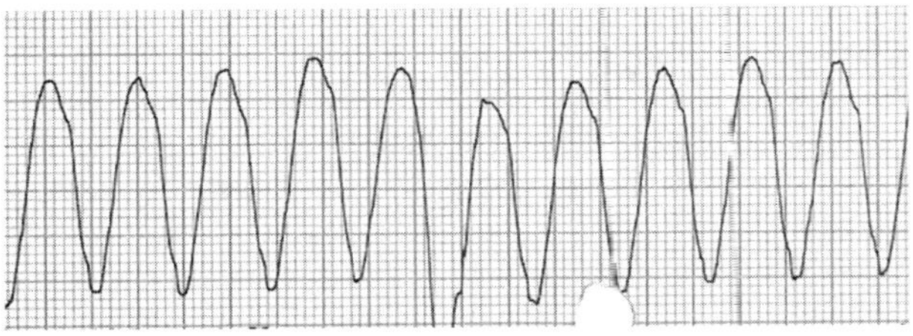

14.

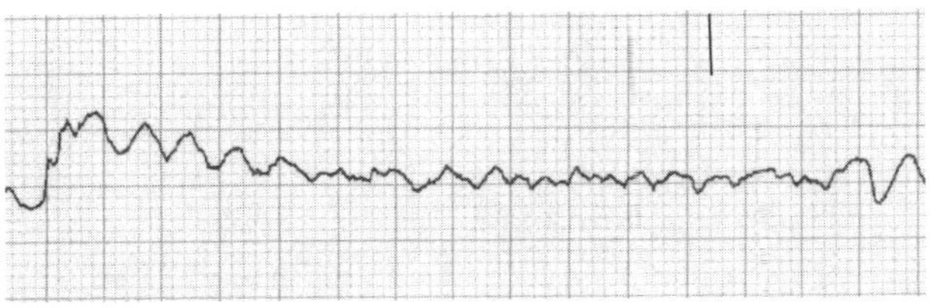

15.

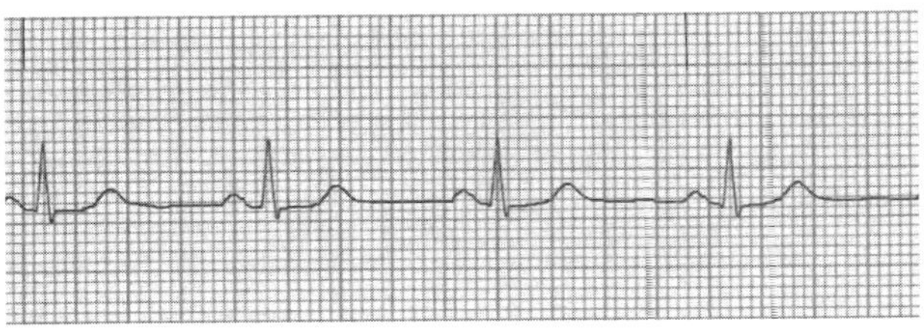

16.

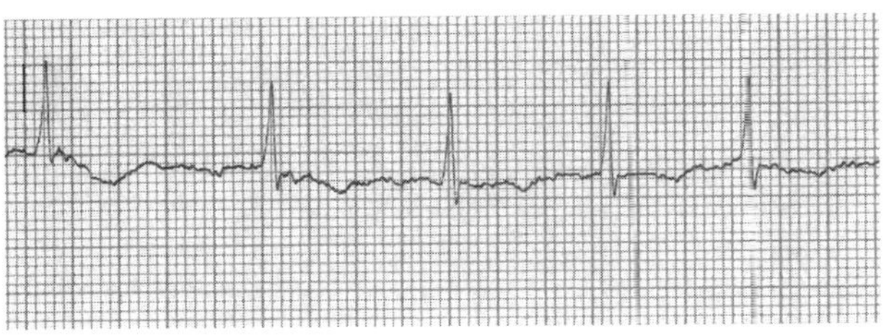

10. Identify potentially lethal EKG changes and describe emergency response

Multiple Choice

1. Why must the MA observe a patient's condition carefully during an EKG?
   (A) It will help him interpret the EKG.
   (B) The provider will expect a report.
   (C) The MA may be the first person to see a change that means emergency care is needed.
   (D) It reassures the patient.

2. Which of the following can be a sign of a cardiac emergency?
   (A) Heart rate of 90
   (B) Deep, regular breathing
   (C) Heart rate of 65
   (D) Sweating

3. As an MA performs an EKG, she sees the tracing suddenly change appearance. What should she do?
   (A) Tell the provider immediately
   (B) Run a diagnostic program on the EKG machine
   (C) Repeat the EKG
   (D) Turn the EKG machine off and then on again

4. An automated external defibrillator can correct some dangerous heart rhythms with
   (A) Medication
   (B) A shock
   (C) Chest compressions
   (D) Rescue breaths

5. AEDs are made to be used by
   (A) Cardiologists
   (B) Any licensed healthcare professional
   (C) EKG technicians and other certified healthcare workers
   (D) Anyone

6. Which of the following lists includes drugs that are commonly given during a cardiac emergency?
   (A) Coumadin, vasopressin, and acetaminophen
   (B) Aspirin, nitroglycerin, and oxygen
   (C) Nitroglycerin, albuterol, and epinephrine
   (D) Labetalol, fluoxetine, and aspirin

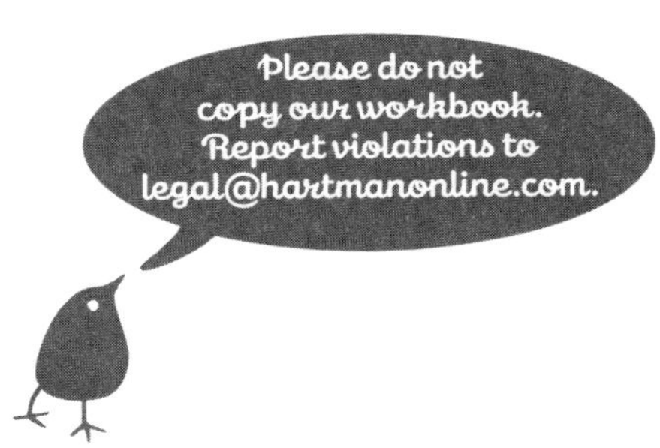

Name: ________________________________

26

Pharmacology and Medication Administration

1. Define *pharmacology* and related terms

Fill in the Blank

1. ______________ is the branch of medicine that studies the uses and effects of drugs.
2. After a drug is administered, it is processed in four stages: ______________, ______________, ______________, and ______________.
3. ______________ is how the drug moves from where it is administered to the bloodstream.
4. ______________ is how the drug moves from the bloodstream to the tissues of the body.
5. ______________ is how the drug is broken down by the body as time passes.
6. ______________ is how the drug leaves the body.

2. Describe drug classes and controlled medications

Short Answer

1. What are a drug's indications?

____

____

2. What are contraindications?

____

____

____

____

3. From your own experience, give an example of a drug that has more than one indication. Name the drug and list at least two indications.

____

____

____

____

4. What do antitussives treat?

____

5. What condition may lead to a prescription for an antihyperlipidemic drug?

____

6. Describe the MA's role in communicating prescriptions to a pharmacy.

____

____

____

____

____

____

7. How are controlled drugs categorized (scheduled)?

____

____

____

____

____

____

8. What is *diversion*? What measures may be in place in a medical office to prevent it?

____

____

____

____

____

____

3. Understand how medications work in the body

True or False

1. ____ Receptors are the parts of cells that receive chemical information.
2. ____ Drugs always work by deactivating receptors.
3. ____ Side effects only happen when a large amount of medication is taken.
4. ____ Side effects are mostly predictable.
5. ____ Systemic side effects can be more serious than local side effects.
6. ____ An idiosyncratic drug reaction is one that is known and expected.
7. ____ If anaphylaxis is going to occur, it always occurs within minutes of the first time a person takes a drug.
8. ____ Immediate response to anaphylaxis can save a person's life.
9. ____ Epinephrine is never administered by anyone other than a licensed medical professional.
10. ____ Signs/symptoms of anaphylaxis include constricted airway, hives, hypotension, and nausea.
11. ____ If, during intake, an MA learns that the patient is taking two drugs that commonly interact, he should tell the patient to stop taking one of them.

Matching

Match each term with the correct example below. Use each letter only once.

12. ____ Local side effect
13. ____ Systemic side effect
14. ____ Hypersensitivity
15. ____ Paradoxical reaction
16. ____ Drug-disease interaction
17. ____ Drug-drug interaction
18. ____ Drug-nutrient interaction

(A) Aspirin can increase bleeding problems in a patient with hemophilia.

(B) Iron supplements may cause constipation.

(C) Anxiolytic drugs may increase anxiety in some patients.

(D) Penicillin may cause hives in some patients.

(E) Dairy products can reduce the effectiveness of some antibiotics.

(F) A COVID-19 booster shot may cause soreness in the arm where it is administered.

(G) Antidepressants and drugs for attention deficit disorder, taken together, can increase the risk of a condition called *serotonin syndrome*.

4. Identify common medication forms and routes of administration

Multiple Choice

1. What is the most common form of medication?
   (A) Syrup
   (B) Tablet
   (C) Spray
   (D) Capsule

2. Which of the following must always be shaken before administration?
   (A) A suspension
   (B) A solution
   (C) A syrup
   (D) A capsule

3. What is the purpose of the groove on a scored tablet?
   (A) It is decorative.
   (B) It is a manufacturer's brand mark.
   (C) It makes the tablet easier to split.
   (D) It makes the tablet easier to crush.

4. If a tablet has an enteric coating or a coating to delay the release of medication, which of the following is true?
   (A) The tablet should not be split or crushed.
   (B) The tablet should be taken with as little liquid as possible.
   (C) The tablet should be dissolved in a food or beverage before administering it.
   (D) The tablet is contraindicated for patients with stomach trouble.

5. How are suppositories administered?
   (A) They are swallowed.
   (B) They are injected with a needle and syringe.
   (C) They are placed in the ear.
   (D) They are inserted into the rectum or vagina.

6. Routes that avoid the digestive tract are called
   (A) Non-oral routes
   (B) Non-GI routes
   (C) Parenteral routes
   (D) Parasympathetic routes

Short Answer

7. What is the difference between an intradermal and a subcutaneous injection?

____

____

____

____

____

8. How is a flu shot usually administered?

____

____

9. What injection route cannot be administered by an MA?

____

10. *Optic*, *ophthalmic*, and *ocular* are all terms that may be used to describe drugs administered to what part of the body?

____

11. Drugs given by the otic route are generally in this form.

____

12. What happens to medications that are administered by the nebulization route?

____

____

____

13. List five forms of medications that may be administered by the topical route.

____

____

____

____

14. What route is commonly used for drugs that must be delivered slowly and continuously for hours or days?

____

5. Discuss measurement of medications and dosage calculation

True or False

1. ____ MAs use household measurements such as teaspoons when administering liquid medications in a healthcare facility.

Name: ____________________

2. ____ When a licensed healthcare professional converts a medication dose, the original prescribed amount in weight or volume must not change.

3. ____ MAs who check dosages before administering a drug may catch an error and prevent harm to a patient.

4. ____ Metric units are based on multiples of 5.

5. ____ In the metric system, weight is measured in ounces and pounds.

6. ____ All states allow MAs to administer medications.

7. ____ A licensed provider may be required to prepare a medication or check dosage before a drug is administered by an MA.

8. ____ The strength of a drug refers to the amount of active ingredient in one unit.

9. ____ Dose and strength are the same thing.

10. ____ Medication orders may list generic or brand names of drugs.

Scenarios

For each scenario, show how the MA would calculate or check the dose to be administered.

11. Arlene reports that she has been experiencing a lot of swelling and her blood pressure has been high. When MA Lalida measures her blood pressure it is 155/102. The provider prescribes 25 mg of the diuretic hydrochlorothiazide orally once daily. She instructs Lalida to administer a dose before Arlene leaves the office. The office's stock of hydrochlorothiazide is in 12.5 mg tablets. How many tablets should Lalida administer?

____

____

____

____

____

12. Simon is an MA in a state that allows him to administer drugs by injection. Agnes is a patient who has been diagnosed with a severe UTI. The provider has ordered an injection of 2 grams of the antibiotic Rocephin (ceftriaxone). The office has 500-mg vials in stock. How many will Simon need to use?

____

____

____

____

____

13. Collette has diabetes. When MA Sonia tests her glucose level it is 220 mg/dL. The provider would like to see it down to 120 mg/dL and orders an insulin injection; 1 unit of insulin should decrease Collette's blood sugar by 50 mg/dL. How many units of insulin will Sonia administer to reach the target of 120 mg/dL?

____

____

____

____

____

6. Discuss safe storage, handling, and disposal of medications

Fill in the blank

1. Medication storage areas should be ____________________ when not in use.

2. Medications that have expired, been contaminated/damaged, or refused after they were prepared must be ____________________ or ____________________.

3. Disposal of any medication must be ____________________ and reported.

4. Medications that are not stored properly may lose their ____________________ or even become ____________________.

5. Most drugs can be stored at ____________ ______________________________.

6. It is a good idea for MAs to know where in the community patients can take prescription drugs for ____________________.

7. Explain the "rights" of medication administration

Matching

Match each medication "right" with an example below. Use each letter only once.

1. ____ Right patient
2. ____ Right medication
3. ____ Right dose
4. ____ Right route
5. ____ Right time
6. ____ Right documentation

(A) A provider asks MA Josiah to administer a medication that is ordered to be taken first thing in the morning, an hour before any food is eaten. It is 8:00 a.m. and Josiah confirms that the patient has not had any food yet.

(B) Olga picked up a new prescription right before coming to an appointment and the provider asks MA Pamela to assist her with taking her first dose. She is prescribed 30 mg/day and has one bottle of 20-mg capsules and one bottle of 10-mg capsules. Pamela instructs her to take one of each.

(C) Ruthie and Natasha, 10-year-old twins, arrived together for a well check. Ruthie recently had her ears pierced. The provider diagnosed cellulitis in the tissue around the piercing and prepared an antibiotic injection, which he assigned MA Dexter to administer. When Dexter enters the exam room he asks Ruthie to state her name and date of birth and confirms with Ruthie's mother.

(D) Iona's asthma has been out of control lately, and during an exam her peak flow is in the yellow range. Her provider asks MA John to administer a dose of prednisone. When he goes to the medication room, John checks closely to make sure he removes the bottle of prednisone and not prednisolone or any other drug.

(E) After administering Ruthie's antibiotic, Dexter enters the medication, dose, route, and time in her EHR.

(F) Zachary is a preschooler who is seen at his pediatrician's office for conjunctivitis. The doctor prescribes antibiotic eyedrops and asks MA Ana to administer the first dose in the office. Ana sees that the antibiotic ordered is in the office's medication room in several forms, including a powder for oral suspension, eyedrops, and eye ointment. She selects the eyedrops.

8. Discuss procedures for medication administration by route

Short Answer

1. What are the three safety checks required before a drug is administered?

____

____

____

____

____

____

2. What is tall man lettering and why might it be used?

____

____

____

____

____

____

Name: ______________________

3. How should a patient be positioned when an oral medication is administered?

____

____

4. Where is a buccal medication placed?

____

____

5. Where is a sublingual medication placed?

____

____

6. What instruction should be given to a patient when a buccal or sublingual medication is administered?

____

____

7. Describe an inhalation chamber/spacer and how it is used.

____

____

____

____

____

____

8. In addition to the medication itself, what may be put in the medication chamber of a nebulizer?

____

9. What may need to be done to prepare a nasal spray for administration?

____

____

10. How should a patient's head be positioned when a nasal spray is administered?

____

____

True or False

11. ____ Gloves are always worn when medications are administered to the eyes.

12. ____ If a second drop of eye medication or a second type of medication is to be administered to the same eye, the MA should wait 1 minute before administering the second drop or medication.

13. ____ Pressing on the middle of the closed eyelid helps ensure that an ophthalmic medication is absorbed.

14. ____ Eye ointment is applied in a thin line to the upper eyelid.

15. ____ After instilling ear drops, the MA should place a clean cotton ball over the ear canal and ask the patient to stay in the same position for 3–5 minutes.

16. ____ Topical medications may be rubbed in or left on the top of the skin.

17. ____ A transdermal medication patch should not be touched with bare hands, even if it is used.

18. ____ When administering medications by the rectal or vaginal routes, privacy and tact are very important.

19. ____ If an MA sees any cracks or rough edges on an applicator for a vaginal medication, she should use the applicator with caution.

20. ____ Suppositories or applicators for rectal or vaginal medications may need to be lubricated.

9. Demonstrate administering medications by injection

Fill in the Blank

1. Needles for injected medications come in a variety of ______________ and ______________.

2. Medications provided in ampules must be drawn up using a needle with a(n) ______________.

3. Powdered injectable drugs must be ________________, or made into liquid form, before they can be administered.

4. When a medication for injection is in powder form, it must be mixed with a liquid called a(n) ____________.

5. Mix a medication for injection carefully by ______________ it in your ____________.

6. After a medication is drawn up in a syringe, the MA must __________ the medication and dose once more with the provider's ____________.

Multiple Choice

7. Which of the following is a common site for an intradermal injection?
   (A) The abdomen
   (B) The inner forearm
   (C) The front of the thigh
   (D) The deltoid

8. What should an MA do with his nondominant hand when preparing to give an intradermal injection?
   (A) Pull the patient's skin taut
   (B) Pinch the skin around the injection site
   (C) Steady the patient
   (D) Brace himself

9. At what angle should the needle be positioned for an intradermal injection?
   (A) 5 degrees
   (B) 10 degrees
   (C) 20 degrees
   (D) 30 degrees

10. What is the most typical angle for administering a subcutaneous injection?
   (A) 10 degrees
   (B) 30 degrees
   (C) 45 degrees
   (D) 90 degrees

11. How should the bevel be positioned for a subcutaneous injection?
   (A) Bevel down
   (B) Bevel to the left
   (C) Bevel to the right
   (D) Bevel up

12. What is the anatomical term for the preferred site for children 3 and under to receive an intramuscular injection?
   (A) *Gluteus maximus*
   (B) *Vastus lateralis*
   (C) Median cubital
   (D) Ventrogluteal

13. How can an MA find the appropriate location for an intramuscular injection in the deltoid?
   (A) It is a full hand width below the shoulder bone.
   (B) It is immediately below the shoulder bone.
   (C) It is 2–3 fingers' width below the shoulder bone.
   (D) It is 2–3 fingers' width above the shoulder bone.

Short Answer

14. Describe the location where IM injections are given in the *vastus lateralis*.

____
____
____
____
____
____
____
____

15. Describe how an MA would find the correct location for a ventrogluteal injection.

____
____
____
____
____
____
____
____

16. How is a Z-track injection administered?

10. List commonly prescribed medications

Short Answer

Choose five of the medications listed in the chart of common drugs on pp. 481–485 in your textbook. For each one, list the name(s) of the medication and describe an imaginary patient who may take the drug. For example, "Lisinopril: Janet is a 50-year-old female with a history of hypertension."

1.

2.

3.

4.

5.

Name: ______________________

Procedure Checklists

Washing hands (hand hygiene)			
	Procedure Steps	yes	no
1.	Turns on water at the sink, keeping clothes dry and away from sink.		
2.	Wets hands and wrists thoroughly.		
3.	Applies soap to hands.		
4.	Keeps hands lower than elbows and fingertips down. Rubs hands together and lathers all surfaces of wrists, fingers, and hands, using friction for at least 20 seconds.		
5.	Cleans nails by rubbing them in the palm of the other hand.		
6.	Keeps hands lower than elbows and fingertips down. Without touching the sink, rinses all surfaces of hands and wrists, running water from wrists to fingertips. Does not run water over unwashed arms down to clean hands.		
7.	Uses clean, dry paper towel to dry all surfaces of hands, wrists, and fingers. Does not wipe towel on unwashed forearms. Discards towel without touching container.		
8.	Uses clean, dry paper towel to turn off faucet, then disposes of paper towel without contaminating hands.		

Date Reviewed ______ Instructor Signature ______

Date Performed ______ Instructor Signature ______

Putting on (donning) and removing (doffing) a gown			
	Procedure Steps	yes	no
1.	Washes hands.		
2.	Opens gown and allows it to open/unfold without shaking it or touching it to floor. Places arms through each sleeve.		
3.	Fastens neck opening.		
4.	Pulls gown until it completely covers clothing. Secures gown at waist.		
5.	Puts on gloves after putting on gown.		
6.	Removes and discards gloves before removing gown. Unfastens gown at waist and neck and removes gown without touching outside of gown. Rolls dirty side in, while holding gown away from body. Discards gown properly and washes hands.		

Date Reviewed ______ Instructor Signature ______

Date Performed ______ Instructor Signature ______

Putting on (donning) a mask and goggles			
	Procedure Steps	yes	no
1.	Washes hands.		
2.	Picks up mask by top strings or elastic strap. Does not touch mask where it touches face.		
3.	Pulls elastic strap over head or ties top strings first then bottom strings.		
4.	Pinches metal strip at top of mask tightly around nose.		

Name: ______________________

5.	Puts on goggles.		
6.	Puts on gloves after putting on mask and goggles.		

Date Reviewed ____________ Instructor Signature ____________

Date Performed ____________ Instructor Signature ____________

Putting on (donning) gloves

	Procedure Steps	yes	no
1.	Washes hands.		
2.	If right-handed, slides one glove on left hand (reverse if left-handed).		
3.	Using gloved hand, slides other hand into second glove.		
4.	Interlaces fingers to smooth out folds and create a comfortable fit.		
5.	Carefully looks for tears, holes, or discolored spots. Replaces glove if needed.		
6.	If wearing a gown, pulls cuffs of gloves over sleeves of gown.		

Date Reviewed ____________ Instructor Signature ____________

Date Performed ____________ Instructor Signature ____________

Removing (doffing) gloves

	Procedure Steps	yes	no
1.	Touches only the outside of one glove and grasps other glove at the palm. Pulls glove off.		
2.	With fingertips of gloved hand, holds removed glove. With ungloved hand, slips two fingers underneath cuff of the remaining glove at wrist without touching any part of the outside.		
3.	Pulls down, turning this glove inside out and over the first glove.		

4.	Discards gloves without contaminating self.		
5.	Washes hands.		

Date Reviewed ____________ Instructor Signature ____________

Date Performed ____________ Instructor Signature ____________

Donning a full set of PPE

	Procedure Steps	yes	no
1.	Washes hands.		
2.	Puts on gown properly.		
3.	Puts on mask or respirator properly.		
4.	Puts on goggles or face shield properly.		
5.	Puts on gloves properly.		

Date Reviewed ____________ Instructor Signature ____________

Date Performed ____________ Instructor Signature ____________

Doffing a full set of PPE

	Procedure Steps	yes	no
1.	Removes and discards gloves properly.		
2.	Removes and discards goggles and face shield properly.		
3.	Removes and discards gown properly.		
4.	Removes and discards mask properly.		
5.	Washes hands.		

Date Reviewed ____________ Instructor Signature ____________

Date Performed ____________ Instructor Signature ____________

Name: ______________________

Performing abdominal thrusts for the conscious person			
	Procedure Steps	yes	no
1.	Stands behind person and brings arms under person's arms. Wraps arms around person's waist.		
2.	Makes a fist with one hand. Places thumb side of the fist against person's abdomen, above the navel but below the breastbone.		
3.	Grasps the fist with other hand. Pulls both hands toward self and up, quickly and forcefully.		
4.	Repeats until the object is pushed out or the person loses consciousness.		
5.	Reports and documents incident properly.		

Date Reviewed ____________ Instructor Signature ____________

Date Performed ____________ Instructor Signature ____________

Responding to shock			
	Procedure Steps	yes	no
1.	Notifies provider immediately.		
2.	Puts on gloves and controls bleeding if bleeding occurs.		
3.	Has the person lie down on her back unless bleeding from the mouth or vomiting. Elevates legs 8 to 12 inches if no signs of injury, breathing difficulties, or fractures exist.		
4.	Checks pulse and respirations if possible. Begins CPR if breathing and pulse are absent, if trained to do so.		
5.	Keeps person as calm and comfortable as possible.		
6.	Maintains normal body temperature.		
7.	Does not give person food or liquids.		
8.	Reports and documents incident properly.		

Date Reviewed ____________ Instructor Signature ____________

Date Performed ____________ Instructor Signature ____________

Responding to a myocardial infarction			
	Procedure Steps	yes	no
1.	Notifies provider immediately.		
2.	Places person in a comfortable position. Encourages him to rest and reassures him that he will not be left alone.		
3.	Loosens clothing around the neck.		
4.	Does not give person liquids or food.		
5.	Monitors person's breathing and pulse. If breathing stops or person has no pulse, performs CPR if trained to do so.		
6.	Stays with person until help arrives.		
7.	Reports and documents incident properly.		

Date Reviewed ____________ Instructor Signature ____________

Date Performed ____________ Instructor Signature ____________

Controlling bleeding			
	Procedure Steps	yes	no
1.	Notifies provider immediately.		
2.	Puts on gloves.		

Name: ______________________

		yes	no
3.	Holds thick pad, clean cloth, or clean towel against wound.		
4.	Presses down hard directly on bleeding wound until help arrives. Does not decrease pressure. Puts additional pads over the first pad if blood seeps through. Does not remove first pad.		
5.	Raises wound above level of heart to slow bleeding.		
6.	When bleeding is under control, secures dressing to keep it in place. Checks for symptoms of shock. Stays with person until help arrives.		
7.	Removes and discards gloves. Washes hands.		
8.	Reports and documents incident properly.		

Date Reviewed ____________ Instructor Signature ____________

Date Performed ____________ Instructor Signature ____________

Treating burns

	Procedure Steps	yes	no
	To treat a minor burn:		
1.	Notifies provider immediately. Puts on gloves.		
2.	Uses cool, clean water to decrease skin temperature and prevent further injury. Does not use ice or ice water, ointment, salve, or grease. Dampens a clean cloth and covers burn.		
3.	Covers area with a dry, clean dressing or nonadhesive sterile bandage.		
4.	Removes and discards gloves. Washes hands.		
	For more serious burns:		
1.	Removes person from source of burn.		
2.	Notifies provider immediately. Puts on gloves.		
3.	Checks for breathing, pulse, and severe bleeding. Begins CPR if trained and allowed to do so.		
4.	Does not use any type of ointment, water, salve, or grease on the burn.		
5.	Does not pull away any clothing from burned areas. Covers burn with sterile gauze or a clean sheet.		
6.	Monitors vital signs and waits for emergency medical help.		
7.	Removes and discards gloves. Washes hands.		
8.	Reports and documents incident properly.		

Date Reviewed ____________ Instructor Signature ____________

Date Performed ____________ Instructor Signature ____________

Responding to fainting

	Procedure Steps	yes	no
1.	Notifies provider immediately.		
2.	Has person lie down or sit down before fainting occurs.		
3.	If person is in a sitting position, has him bend forward and place his head between his knees if he is able. If person is lying flat on his back, elevates his legs about 12 inches.		
4.	Loosens any tight clothing.		
5.	Has person stay in position for at least 5 minutes after symptoms disappear.		
6.	Helps person get up slowly. Continues to observe him for symptoms of fainting.		

Name: ______________________

7.	If person faints, lowers him to floor and positions him on his back. Elevates his legs 8 to 12 inches if no sign of injury, breathing difficulties, or fractures. Checks for breathing.		
8.	Reports and documents incident properly.		

______ Date Reviewed ______ Instructor Signature

______ Date Performed ______ Instructor Signature

Responding to nosebleed

	Procedure Steps	yes	no
1.	Notifies provider immediately.		
2.	Tells person to remain sitting, leaning forward slightly. Offers tissues or a clean cloth.		
3.	Puts on gloves. Applies firm pressure on both sides of nose, on the soft part, up near bridge. Squeezes sides of nose with thumb and forefinger.		
4.	Applies pressure until bleeding stops.		
5.	Uses a cool cloth or ice wrapped in a cloth on bridge of nose to slow blood flow.		
6.	Removes and discards gloves. Washes hands.		
7.	Reports and documents incident properly.		

______ Date Reviewed ______ Instructor Signature

______ Date Performed ______ Instructor Signature

Responding to a seizure

	Procedure Steps	yes	no
1.	Notes the time and puts on gloves.		
2.	Lowers person to floor. Tries to turn person to one side to help lower risk of choking.		
3.	Has someone call provider immediately. Does not leave person unless to get medical help.		
4.	Moves furniture away.		
5.	Does not try to restrain the person.		
6.	Does not force anything between the person's teeth. Does not place hands in person's mouth.		
7.	Does not give food or liquids.		
8.	When the seizure is over, notes time and turns person on left side if injury is not suspected. Checks breathing and pulse. Begins CPR if breathing and pulse are absent and if trained and allowed to do so.		
9.	Removes and discards gloves. Washes hands.		
10.	Reports and documents incident properly.		

______ Date Reviewed ______ Instructor Signature

______ Date Performed ______ Instructor Signature

Responding to vomiting

	Procedure Steps	yes	no
1.	Notifies provider immediately.		
2.	Puts on gloves.		
3.	Makes sure patient's head is up or turned to one side. Places emesis basin under chin and removes it when vomiting has stopped.		
4.	Assists patient to clean up.		

Name: ______________________

5.	Flushes vomit down toilet unless vomit is red, has blood in it, or looks like wet coffee grounds. Places disposable basin in biohazardous waste container or disinfects reusable basin.		
6.	Removes and discards gloves.		
7.	Washes hands.		
8.	Puts on clean gloves.		
9.	Provides comfort to patient.		
10.	Puts soiled linens in proper container.		
11.	Removes and discards gloves.		
12.	Washes hands again.		
13.	Documents time, amount, color, and consistency of vomitus.		

Date Reviewed	Instructor Signature
Date Performed	Instructor Signature

Measuring and recording an oral temperature

	Procedure Steps	yes	no
1.	Identifies self by name. Identifies patient.		
2.	Washes hands.		
3.	Explains procedure to patient, speaking clearly, slowly, and directly. Maintains face-to-face contact whenever possible.		
4.	Puts on gloves.		
5.	**Digital thermometer:** Puts on disposable sheath. Turns on thermometer and waits until ready sign appears.		
	Electronic thermometer: Removes probe from base unit and puts on probe cover.		
	Mercury-free thermometer: Holds thermometer by stem. Shakes thermometer down to below the lowest number.		
6.	**Digital thermometer:** Inserts end of digital thermometer into patient's mouth, under tongue and to one side.		
	Electronic thermometer: Inserts end of electronic thermometer into patient's mouth, under tongue and to one side.		
	Mercury-free thermometer: Puts on a disposable sheath. Inserts bulb end of thermometer into patient's mouth, under tongue and to one side.		
7.	**For all thermometers:** Tells patient how to hold thermometer in mouth.		
	Digital thermometer: Holds in place until thermometer blinks or beeps.		
	Electronic thermometer: Holds in place until tone or light signals temperature has been read.		
	Mercury-free thermometer: Holds in place for at least 3 minutes.		
8.	**Digital thermometer:** Removes thermometer. Reads temperature on display screen. Remembers temperature reading.		
	Electronic thermometer: Reads temperature on display screen. Remembers temperature reading. Removes probe.		
	Mercury-free thermometer: Removes thermometer. Wipes with tissue from stem to bulb or removes sheath. Discards tissue or sheath. Reads temperature and remembers reading.		

Name: ______________________________

9.	**Digital thermometer:** Removes and discards sheath. Replaces thermometer in case.		
	Electronic thermometer: Presses eject button to discard cover. Returns probe to holder.		
	Mercury-free thermometer: Cleans thermometer according to office guidelines. Rinses and dries thermometer. Returns to case.		
10.	Removes and discards gloves. Washes hands.		
11.	Immediately records temperature, date, time, and method used.		
12.	Reports any changes in pat ent to provider.		

Date Reviewed ______ Instructor Signature ______

Date Performed ______ Instructor Signature ______

Measuring and recording a rectal temperature			
	Procedure Steps	yes	no
1.	Identifies self by name. Identifies patient.		
2.	Washes hands.		
3.	Explains procedure to patient, speaking clearly, slowly, and directly. Maintains face-to-face contact whenever possible.		
4.	Instructs patient to remove necessary clothing. Provides patient with covering for privacy.		
5.	Helps patient to left-lying position.		
6.	Folds back covering to expose only rectal area.		
7.	Puts on gloves.		
8.	**Digital thermometer**: Puts on disposable sheath. Turns on thermometer and waits until ready sign appears.		
	Electronic thermometer: Removes probe from base unit. Puts on probe cover.		
	Mercury-free thermometer: Holds thermometer by stem. Shakes thermometer down to below lowest number. Puts on disposable sheath.		
9.	Applies a small amount of lubricant (if sheath not prelubricated).		
10.	Separates buttocks. Gently inserts thermometer into rectum ½ to 1 inch.		
11.	Replaces sheet over buttocks. Holds on to thermometer at all times.		
12.	**Digital thermometer:** Holds in place until thermometer blinks or beeps.		
	Electronic thermometer: Holds in place until tone or light signals temperature has been read.		
	Mercury-free thermometer: Holds in place for at least 3 minutes.		
13.	Gently removes thermometer. Wipes with tissue from stem to bulb or removes sheath. Discards tissue or sheath.		
14.	Reads thermometer and remembers reading.		
15.	**Digital thermometer:** Cleans thermometer according to facility guidelines. Replaces thermometer in case.		
	Electronic thermometer: Presses eject button to discard cover. Returns probe to holder.		
	Mercury-free thermometer: Cleans thermometer according to facility guidelines. Rinses and dries thermometer. Returns to case.		
16.	Removes and discards gloves.		

Name: ______________________

17.	Assists patient to a position of safety and comfort.		
18.	Washes hands.		
19.	Immediately records temperature, date, time, and method used.		
20.	Removes privacy measures.		
21.	Reports any changes in patient to provider.		

Date Reviewed ______ Instructor Signature ______

Date Performed ______ Instructor Signature ______

Measuring and recording a tympanic temperature

	Procedure Steps	yes	no
1.	Identifies self by name. Identifies patient.		
2.	Washes hands.		
3.	Explains procedure to patient, speaking clearly, slowly, and directly. Maintains face-to-face contact whenever possible.		
4.	Puts on gloves.		
5.	Puts disposable sheath over earpiece of thermometer.		
6.	Positions patient's head and pulls up and back on outside edge of ear for adult, down and back for child. Inserts covered probe and presses button.		
7.	Holds thermometer in place until it blinks or beeps.		
8.	Reads temperature and remembers reading.		
9.	Disposes of sheath. Returns thermometer to storage or to battery charger if thermometer is rechargeable.		
10.	Removes and discards gloves. Washes hands.		
11.	Immediately records temperature, date, time, and method used.		
12.	Reports any changes in patient to provider.		

Date Reviewed ______ Instructor Signature ______

Date Performed ______ Instructor Signature ______

Measuring and recording an axillary temperature

	Procedure Steps	yes	no
1.	Identifies self by name. Identifies patient.		
2.	Washes hands.		
3.	Explains procedure to patient, speaking clearly, slowly, and directly. Maintains face-to-face contact whenever possible.		
4.	Puts on gloves.		
5.	Asks patient to remove clothing for skin contact with end of thermometer. Wipes axillary area with tissues.		
6.	**Digital thermometer:** Puts on disposable sheath. Turns on thermometer and waits until ready sign appears.		
	Electronic thermometer: Removes probe from base unit. Puts on probe cover.		
	Mercury-free thermometer: Holds thermometer by stem. Shakes down below lowest number. Puts on disposable sheath.		
7.	Positions thermometer (bulb end for mercury-free) in center of armpit. Folds patient's arm over his chest.		
8.	**Digital thermometer:** Holds in place until thermometer blinks or beeps.		

	Electronic thermometer: Holds in place until a tone is heard or a flashing or steady light is seen.		
	Mercury-free thermometer: Holds in place, with arm close against side, for 8 to 10 minutes.		
9.	**Digital thermometer:** Removes thermometer. Reads temperature and remembers reading.		
	Electronic thermometer: Reads temperature and remembers reading. Removes probe.		
	Mercury-free thermometer: Removes thermometer. Wipes with a tissue from stem to bulb or removes sheath. Discards tissue or sheath. Reads temperature and remembers reading.		
10.	**Digital thermometer:** Removes and discards sheath. Replaces thermometer in case.		
	Electronic thermometer: Presses eject button to discard cover. Returns probe to holder.		
	Mercury-free thermometer: Cleans thermometer according to facility guidelines. Rinses and dries thermometer. Returns to case.		
11.	Removes and discards gloves.		
12.	Immediately records temperature, date, time, and method used.		
13.	Assists patient to replace clothing as needed.		
14.	Washes hands.		
15.	Reports any changes in patient to provider.		

Date Reviewed ______ Instructor Signature ______

Date Performed ______ Instructor Signature ______

Counting and recording apical pulse

	Procedure Steps	yes	no
1.	Identifies self by name. Identifies patient.		
2.	Washes hands.		
3.	Explains procedure to patient, speaking clearly, slowly, and directly. Maintains face-to-face contact whenever possible.		
4.	Before using stethoscope, wipes diaphragm and earpieces with alcohol wipes.		
5.	Fits earpieces of stethoscope snugly in ears and places flat metal diaphragm on left side of chest, just below nipple. Listens for heartbeat.		
6.	Counts heartbeats for 1 minute.		
7.	Washes hands.		
8.	Immediately records pulse rate, date, time, and method used. Notes any irregularities in rhythm.		
9.	Cleans earpieces and diaphragm of stethoscope. Stores stethoscope.		
10.	Washes hands.		
11.	Reports to provider if pulse is less than 60 beats per minute, over 100 beats per minute, if rhythm is irregular, or if breathing is irregular.		

Date Reviewed ______ Instructor Signature ______

Date Performed ______ Instructor Signature ______

Counting and recording radial pulse and counting and recording respirations

	Procedure Steps	yes	no
1.	Identifies self by name. Identifies patient.		

Name: ______________________________

2.	Washes hands.		
3.	Explains procedure to patient, speaking clearly, slowly, and directly. Maintains face-to-face contact whenever possible.		
4.	Places tips of index finger and middle finger on thumb side of patient's wrist to locate radial pulse.		
5.	Counts beats for 1 full minute.		
6.	Keeps fingertips on patient's wrist and counts respirations for 1 full minute.		
7.	Washes hands.		
8.	Immediately records pulse rate, date, time, and method used. Records respiratory rate and pattern or character of breathing.		
9.	Reports to provider if pulse is less than 60 beats per minute, over 100 beats per minute, if rhythm is irregular, or if breathing is irregular.		

______________ Date Reviewed ______________ Instructor Signature

______________ Date Performed ______________ Instructor Signature

Measuring and recording a pulse oximetry reading

	Procedure Steps	yes	no
1.	Identifies self by name. Identifies patient.		
2.	Washes hands.		
3.	Explains procedure to patient, speaking clearly, slowly, and directly. Maintains face-to-face contact whenever possible.		
4.	Chooses proper sensor.		
5.	Identifies site for sensor and removes nail polish if needed.		
6.	Places sensor on proper site.		
7.	Instructs patient to keep sensor in place until reading is displayed.		
8.	Washes hands.		
9.	Records reading.		
10.	Reports abnormal reading to provider.		

______________ Date Reviewed ______________ Instructor Signature

______________ Date Performed ______________ Instructor Signature

Measuring and recording blood pressure manually

	Procedure Steps	yes	no
1.	Identifies self by name. Identifies patient.		
2.	Washes hands.		
3.	Explains procedure to patient, speaking clearly, slowly, and directly. Maintains face-to-face contact whenever possible.		
4.	Wipes diaphragm and earpieces of stethoscope with alcohol wipes.		
5.	Asks patient to roll up sleeve.		
6.	Positions patient's arm palm up and level with the heart.		
7.	With valve open, squeezes cuff to completely deflate.		
8.	Places blood pressure cuff snugly on patient's upper arm, with sensor/arrow over brachial artery.		
9.	Asks patient to remain still and quiet during measurement.		
10.	Locates brachial pulse with fingertips.		
11.	Places earpieces of stethoscope in ears.		

12.	Places diaphragm of stethoscope over brachial artery.		
13.	Closes valve until it stops. Does not overtighten it.		
14.	Inflates cuff to between 160 mm Hg and 180 mm Hg. If beat is heard immediately upon deflation, completely deflates cuff. Reinflates cuff to no more than 200 mm Hg.		
15.	Opens valve slightly with thumb and index finger. Deflates cuff slowly.		
16.	Watches gauge and listens for sound of pulse.		
17.	Remembers reading at which first pulse sound is heard (systolic pressure).		
18.	Continues listening for a change or muffling of pulse sound. Remembers reading at this point (diastolic pressure).		
19.	Opens valve to deflate cuff completely. Removes cuff.		
20.	Washes hands.		
21.	Immediately records systolic and diastolic pressures. Notes which arm was used.		
22.	Cleans stethoscope. Stores equipment.		
23.	Washes hands.		
24.	Reports any changes in patient to provider.		

Date Reviewed ____________ Instructor Signature ____________

Date Performed ____________ Instructor Signature ____________

Measuring and recording blood pressure electronically

	Procedure Steps	yes	no
1.	Identifies self by name. Identifies patient.		
2.	Washes hands.		
3.	Explains procedure to patient, speaking clearly, slowly, and directly. Maintains face-to-face contact whenever possible.		
4.	Asks patient to roll up sleeve.		
5.	Positions patient's arm palm up and level with the heart.		
6.	Makes sure cuff is completely deflated and places cuff snugly on patient's upper arm with sensor/arrow over brachial artery.		
7.	Asks patient to remain still and quiet during measurement.		
8.	Turns on blood pressure device and presses start button.		
9.	Watches for reading to appear on screen.		
10.	Removes cuff.		
11.	Washes hands.		
12.	Immediately records systolic and diastolic pressures. Notes which arm was used.		
13.	Stores equipment.		
14.	Washes hands.		
15.	Reports any changes in patient to provider.		

Date Reviewed ____________ Instructor Signature ____________

Date Performed ____________ Instructor Signature ____________

Measuring and recording weight of an ambulatory patient

	Procedure Steps	yes	no
1.	Identifies self by name. Identifies patient.		
2.	Washes hands.		

Name: ______________________________

		yes	no
3.	Explains procedure to patient, speaking clearly, slowly, and directly. Maintains face-to-face contact whenever possible.		
4.	Starts with scale balanced at 0 (zero).		
5.	Asks patient to step onto center of scale, assisting if needed. Makes sure patient is not holding, touching, or leaning against anything.		
6.	Determines patient's weight.		
7.	Helps patient off scale before recording weight.		
8.	Washes hands.		
9.	Immediately records weight.		
10.	Reports any changes in an established patient's weight to provider.		

Date Reviewed ______ Instructor Signature ______

Date Performed ______ Instructor Signature ______

Measuring and recording weight of an infant

	Procedure Steps	yes	no
1.	Identifies self by name. Identifies patient.		
2.	Washes hands.		
3.	Explains procedure to parent/caregiver, speaking clearly, slowly, and directly. Maintains face-to-face contact whenever possible.		
4.	Starts with scale balanced at 0 (zero). If infant is weighed in a diaper, diaper is added to scale before balancing.		
5.	Removes infant's clothing.		
6.	Places infant in center of scale, protecting sides. Keeps at least one hand near baby.		
7.	Determines patient's weight.		
8.	Removes infant from scale.		
9.	Washes hands.		
10.	Immediately records patient's weight.		
11.	Replaces infant's clothing.		
12.	Reports any significant weight loss or gain to provider.		

Date Reviewed ______ Instructor Signature ______

Date Performed ______ Instructor Signature ______

Measuring and recording height of an ambulatory patient

	Procedure Steps	yes	no
1.	Identifies self by name. Identifies patient.		
2.	Washes hands.		
3.	Explains procedure to patient, speaking clearly, slowly, and directly. Maintains face-to-face contact whenever possible.		
4.	Helps patient step onto scale, facing away from scale.		
5.	Asks patient to stand straight. Helps as needed.		
6.	Pulls up measuring rod from back of scale. Gently lowers rod until it rests flat on patient's head.		
7.	Determines patient's height.		
8.	Helps patient off scale before recording height.		
9.	Washes hands.		
10.	Immediately records patient's height.		

Name: ____________________

11.	Documents procedure using facility guidelines.		

Date Reviewed	Instructor Signature
Date Performed	Instructor Signature

Sanitizing and disinfecting the examination room and instruments

	Procedure Steps	yes	no
1.	Puts on rubber gloves, mask, gown or apron, and eye protection.		
2.	Cleans examination room surfaces with bactericidal solution.		
3.	Places contaminated instruments in bactericidal solution for 10 minutes. Covers them completely with liquid.		
4.	Removes instruments from bactericide and rinses thoroughly in water.		
5.	Uses a scrub brush to remove any remaining contaminant. Rinses thoroughly.		
6.	Places instruments on a sterile field to dry. Scissors and hinged instruments placed in open position.		

Date Reviewed	Instructor Signature
Date Performed	Instructor Signature

Performing sterile wrapping

	Procedure Steps	yes	no
1.	Washes hands.		
2.	Selects a surgical wrap large enough to cover instruments.		
3.	Places wrap on a clean surface in shape of a diamond.		
4.	Places item(s) properly in center of wrap. Scissors and hinged instruments placed in open position.		
5.	Places a sterilization indicator on top of instruments if used.		
6.	Folds bottom side of surgical wrap up snugly. Makes tab at top as instructed.		
7.	Folds left side of wrap over snugly.		
8.	Folds right side of wrap over snugly.		
9.	Folds top down snugly and tucks into envelope created by side folds.		
10.	Folds back corner to form tab for opening.		
11.	Applies autoclave tape to secure package.		
12.	Writes date and initials on tape with permanent marker.		

Date Reviewed	Instructor Signature
Date Performed	Instructor Signature

Performing a sterile hand scrub

	Procedure Steps	yes	no
1.	Removes all jewelry.		
2.	Opens surgical scrub brush package.		
3.	Turns on faucet and adjusts water temperature to warm.		
4.	Applies surgical soap to skin generously. Uses scrub brush to produce a lather.		
5.	Performs a 5-minute scrub, keeping fingers pointed upward. Scrubs one hand thoroughly. Always moves away from fingertips.		

Name: ______________________

6.	Repeats this procedure with remaining hand for a minimum of 5 minutes.		
7.	Rinses thoroughly from fingers to wrists with fingers pointing upward.		
8.	Turns off faucet without touching it with scrubbed hands.		
9.	Pats hands dry with sterile towel. Moves from fingertips to forearms.		
10.	Keeps hands pointed upward, above waist, and in front of body.		

Date Reviewed ______ Instructor Signature ______

Date Performed ______ Instructor Signature ______

Donning sterile gloves

	Procedure Steps	yes	no
1.	Performs a surgical scrub.		
2.	Removes outer packaging of sterile gloves. Places inner package on clean surface.		
3.	Grasps edges of package. Pulls out each side to expose gloves. Does not touch other surfaces of package.		
4.	Grasps one glove at fold along bottom of cuff with nondominant hand.		
5.	Inserts dominant hand into first glove. Does not touch outside of glove.		
6.	Inserts fingers of gloved hand under folded cuff of second glove. Touches only outer surface of glove. Takes care not to touch glove with thumb.		
7.	Inserts ungloved hand into second glove. Takes care not to touch outside of glove.		
8.	Keeps gloved hands above waist and in front of body.		

Date Reviewed ______ Instructor Signature ______

Date Performed ______ Instructor Signature ______

Preparing the sterile field

	Procedure Steps	yes	no
1.	Washes hands. Puts on nonsterile gloves.		
2.	Places Mayo stand cover over Mayo stand. Touches only outer edges of cover.		
3.	Obtains sterile procedure tray. Checks sterilization and expiration dates.		
4.	Places tray on Mayo stand with opening tab facing self.		
5.	Unwraps tray properly. Works from sides and does not lean over a sterile field.		
6.	Performs a sterile scrub. Puts on sterile gloves.		
7.	Arranges sterile items in order of use. Places sharp instruments such as scalpels in easily visible locations on field. Does not use outer 2 inches of field.		
8.	Positions bowls for liquids on edge of sterile field.		
9.	Pours out small amount of any solutions to decontaminate container rim before pouring into sterile bowls.		
10.	Gets any other items needed for procedure. Adds them to sterile field by drop method or with sterile forceps.		

11.	Covers sterile field with sterile towel until ready for use.		
12.	Removes and discards gloves. Washes hands.		

Date Reviewed ____ Instructor Signature ____

Date Performed ____ Instructor Signature ____

Preparing the skin for a surgical procedure

	Procedure Steps	yes	no
1.	Identifies self by name. Identifies patient.		
2.	Explains procedure to patient, speaking clearly, slowly, and directly. Maintains face-to-face contact whenever possible.		
3.	Washes hands.		
4.	If using a skin preparation kit, opens kit and prepares included items as directed. Otherwise, opens sponges and places them on a sterile towel. Saturates half of sponges with first cleaning agent and other half with second agent.		
5.	Performs surgical hand scrub. Puts on sterile gloves.		
6.	One at a time, applies sponges with first agent to operative site. Works outward in a circular motion with friction. Covers an area extending 2" (5 cm) beyond operative site. Discards each sponge after use.		
7.	Continues cleaning with first agent for 2–3 minutes.		
8.	Allows site to air-dry.		
9.	Repeats steps with second agent, cleaning for 2–3 minutes.		
10.	Always moves outward from operative site. Discards sponges after use.		
11.	Allows site to air-dry before draping.		
12.	Removes and discards gloves. Washes hands.		
13.	Reports to provider that patient has been prepared for procedure.		

Date Reviewed ____ Instructor Signature ____

Date Performed ____ Instructor Signature ____

Applying a sterile dressing

	Procedure Steps	yes	no
1.	Identifies self by name. Identifies patient.		
2.	Washes hands.		
3.	Explains procedure to patient, speaking clearly, slowly, and directly. Maintains face-to-face contact whenever possible.		
4.	Opens dressing tray on a clean surface close to site of dressing change.		
5.	Performs a surgical hand scrub. Puts on sterile gloves.		
6.	Cleans surgical wound with antiseptic wipe. Moves from incision outward. Allows incision to air-dry.		
7.	Applies gauze pads to cover incision. Secures dressing with tape.		
8.	Records time and date of dressing on tape.		
9.	Removes and discards gloves. Washes hands.		
10.	Documents appearance of wound and dressing procedure using facility guidelines.		

Date Reviewed ____ Instructor Signature ____

Date Performed ____ Instructor Signature ____

Name: ______________________

Removing sutures or staples			
	Procedure Steps	yes	no
1.	Identifies self by name. Identifies patient.		
2.	Washes hands.		
3.	Explains procedure to patient, speaking clearly, slowly, and directly. Maintains face-to-face contact whenever possible.		
4.	Puts on gloves.		
5.	Removes any dressings.		
6.	Observes wound for drainage, redness, and skin approximation.		
7.	Cleans area with antiseptic wipes.		
8.	Removes and discards gloves.		
9.	Opens suture or staple removal kit.		
10.	Performs surgical hand scrub. Puts on sterile gloves.		
11.	Places gauze next to surgical wound.		
12.	Works from one end of incision to opposite end. Removes each suture or staple.		
	For sutures:		
13.	Grasps suture knot with forceps. Gently lifts knot and slips scissors under suture.		
14.	Clips suture beside knot. Gently slips up to remove. Places each removed suture on gauze.		
	For staples:		
13.	Slips lower end of staple remover under middle of staple. Squeezes handles together firmly.		
14.	Tilts staple remover slightly. Gently lifts up on staple to remove it from skin. Places each removed staple on gauze.		
	Ending steps:		
15.	Cleans site with antiseptic and allows it to air-dry.		
16.	Applies skin closure bandages across wound.		
17.	Discards trash.		
18.	Removes and discards gloves. Washes hands.		
19.	Documents procedure using facility guidelines.		

______________ Date Reviewed ______________ Instructor Signature

______________ Date Performed ______________ Instructor Signature

Assisting with ambulation for a patient using a cane, walker, or crutches			
	Procedure Steps	yes	no
1.	Identifies self by name. Identifies patient.		
2.	Washes hands.		
3.	Explains procedure to patient, speaking clearly, slowly, and directly. Maintains face-to-face contact whenever possible.		
4.	Stands in front of patient with feet about shoulder-width apart. Bends knees. Keeps back straight.		
5.	Places transfer belt around patient's waist over clothing. Grasps belt on both sides with hands in an upward position.		
6.	If patient is unable to stand without help, uses a mechanical lift, if available, or braces patient's lower extremities. Keeps back straight. Helps patient to stand.		
7.	Helps as needed with ambulation with cane, walker, or crutches.		

8.	Walks slightly behind and to one side of patient while holding on to transfer belt.		
9.	Watches for obstacles in patient's path.		
10.	Lets patient set pace, encouraging rest if tired.		
11.	After ambulation, returns patient to a chair or exam table and removes transfer belt.		
12.	Washes hands.		
13.	Documents procedure using facility guidelines.		

Date Reviewed ____________ Instructor Signature ____________

Date Performed ____________ Instructor Signature ____________

Assisting with cast application

	Procedure Steps	yes	no
1.	Identifies self by name. Identifies patient.		
2.	Washes hands.		
3.	Explains procedure to patient, speaking clearly, slowly, and directly. Maintains face-to-face contact whenever possible.		
4.	Asks patient to remove clothing to expose area. Assists if needed.		
5.	Cleans skin and allows it to air-dry.		
6.	Measures site and cuts stockinette 4 inches (10 cm) longer than measurement. Applies stockinette to site, leaving 2 inches (5 cm) of extra fabric at each end.		
7.	Applies padding material around cast area in a spiral motion. Applies extra padding over bony areas.		
8.	Puts on gloves. Completely immerses fiberglass rolls in water basin.		
9.	Assists provider as needed during application of fiberglass rolls.		
10.	Discards any trash.		
11.	Removes and discards gloves. Washes hands.		
12.	Documents procedure using facility guidelines.		

Date Reviewed ____________ Instructor Signature ____________

Date Performed ____________ Instructor Signature ____________

Assisting with lumbar puncture

	Procedure Steps	yes	no
1.	Identifies self by name. Identifies patient.		
2.	Washes hands.		
3.	Explains procedure to patient, speaking clearly, slowly, and directly. Maintains face-to-face contact whenever possible.		
4.	Gives patient a gown and drape. Instructs patient on removal of clothing. Provides privacy.		
5.	After patient has changed, assists them to side-lying position with knees drawn up to chest.		
6.	If assisting with procedure, puts on sterile gown and gloves.		
7.	Cleans injection site and around site (approximately 6 inches or 15 cm) with an antiseptic if directed.		
8.	Assists provider during procedure and monitors patient as directed.		
9.	Removes and discards gloves. Washes hands.		

Name: ______________________

10.	Assists patient to supine position. Has patient lie flat for 20–30 minutes.		
11.	Offers fluids to replace CSF that was removed. Continues to monitor patient.		
12.	Helps patient to sit up. Observes for discomfort.		
13.	Documents patient's response to procedure and recovery using facility guidelines.		

Date Reviewed ______ Instructor Signature ______

Date Performed ______ Instructor Signature ______

Performing vision screening exams

	Procedure Steps	yes	no
1.	Identifies self by name. Identifies patient.		
2.	Washes hands.		
3.	Explains procedure to patient, speaking clearly, slowly, and directly. Maintains face-to-face contact whenever possible.		
4.	Positions patient 20 feet away from Snellen eye chart.		
5.	Asks patient to read first line with both eyes. Moves down chart until patient cannot read a line without 2 or more errors.		
6.	Records results in patient's record.		
7.	Asks patient to use occluder to cover right eye.		
8.	Follows procedure above to measure acuity of left eye. Records results.		
9.	Asks patient to switch occluder to left eye. Repeats procedure. Records results for right eye.		
10.	Tests near vision using a near vision chart. Has patient hold chart about 14 inches (36 cm) in front of them.		
11.	Asks patient to read smallest line that they can see. Notes smallest line that they can read without making an error.		
12.	Obtains Ishihara color plates. Holds them approximately 14 inches (36 cm) in front of patient.		
13.	Asks patient to identify number on each plate. Records number of plates that patient could detect and which ones he could not see.		
14.	Disinfects reusable equipment. Washes hands.		
15.	Documents results using facility guidelines.		

Date Reviewed ______ Instructor Signature ______

Date Performed ______ Instructor Signature ______

Testing hearing acuity with an audiometer

	Procedure Steps	yes	no
1.	Identifies self by name. Identifies patient.		
2.	Washes hands.		
3.	Explains procedure to patient, speaking clearly, slowly, and directly. Maintains face-to-face contact whenever possible.		
4.	Helps patient to put on headphones.		
5.	Tells patient that he will hear sounds in left ear and should raise his hand to indicate when he hears a sound.		

6.	Tests volume of sound. Maintains volume at that level.		
7.	Sets audiometer to lowest frequency to emit sounds in left ear. Emits sound in left ear and observes patient's response.		
8.	Increases frequency one level at a time until patient responds that he can hear tone. Continues to increase frequencies. Records result for each tone.		
9.	Sets audiometer to emit sounds in right ear and repeats test. Records result for each tone.		
10.	Disinfects reusable equipment. Discards any single-use supplies.		
11.	Documents results using facility guidelines.		

Date Reviewed ______________ Instructor Signature ______________

Date Performed ______________ Instructor Signature ______________

Irrigating eyes or ears

	Procedure Steps	yes	no
1.	Identifies self by name. Identifies patient.		
2.	Washes hands.		
3.	Explains procedure to patient, speaking clearly, slowly, and directly. Maintains face-to-face contact whenever possible.		
4.	Puts on gloves.		
	For eye irrigation:		
5.	Places patient upright or in Fowler's position with head tilted toward side to be irrigated.		
6.	Drapes towel over patient's shoulder. Holds emesis basin under eye or has patient hold it.		
7.	Pours irrigating solution into sterile basin. Draws up solution.		
8.	Aims syringe at inner canthus and instills solution.		
9.	Refills syringe and repeats procedure.		
10.	Gives patient a tissue to dry eye when irrigation is complete.		
	For ear irrigation:		
5.	Has patient sit or lie down. Drapes a towel over patient's shoulder.		
6.	Pours irrigating solution into sterile basin. Draws up solution in syringe.		
7.	Asks patient to hold basin below ear. Pulls ear upward.		
8.	Aims syringe at upper edge of ear canal. Slowly instills solution. Allows it to drain out into basin.		
9.	Refills syringe and repeats procedure.		
10.	Dries ear canal when irrigation is complete.		
	For both forms of irrigation:		
11.	Disinfects reusable equipment. Discards trash.		
12.	Removes gloves and washes hands.		
13.	Documents procedure using facility guidelines.		

Date Reviewed ______________ Instructor Signature ______________

Date Performed ______________ Instructor Signature ______________

Performing pulmonary function tests

	Procedure Steps	yes	no
1.	Identifies self by name. Identifies patient.		
2.	Washes hands.		

Name: ____________________

3.	Explains procedure to patient, speaking clearly, slowly, and directly. Maintains face-to-face contact whenever possible.		
4.	Measures patient's height and weight and enters necessary information into spirometer.		
5.	Puts on gloves.		
6.	Assists patient to a seated position. Instructs her to keep her back and neck upright and straight.		
7.	Puts a mouthpiece on spirometer.		
8.	Demonstrates proper procedure to patient.		
9.	Removes and discards mouthpiece.		
10.	Removes gloves. Washes hands.		
11.	Puts on clean gloves.		
12.	Attaches a new mouthpiece to spirometer.		
13.	Applies nose clip to patient's nose. Instructs her how to properly seal mouth around mouthpiece.		
14.	Instructs patient to take deepest breath possible through mouth, seal mouth onto mouthpiece, and exhale with as much force as possible.		
15.	Coaches patient to keep exhaling or blowing out as long as possible.		
16.	Checks spirometer to see if measurement was recorded and accepted.		
17.	Has patient repeat test until three acceptable measurements are obtained.		
18.	Disinfects equipment and discards disposable supplies.		
19.	Removes and discards gloves. Washes hands.		
20.	Documents procedure using facility guidelines.		

Date Reviewed ____________ Instructor Signature ____________

Date Performed ____________ Instructor Signature ____________

Measuring peak expiratory flow rate using a peak flow meter

	Procedure Steps	yes	no
1.	Identifies self by name. Identifies patient.		
2.	Washes hands.		
3.	Explains procedure to patient, speaking clearly, slowly, and directly. Maintains face-to-face contact whenever possible.		
4.	Puts on gloves.		
5.	Asks patient to stand or sit upright.		
6.	Moves marker on meter to lowest setting.		
7.	Instructs patient to take a deep breath, seal lips around mouthpiece, and blow out as hard and fast as possible.		
8.	Makes a note of position of marker.		
9.	Repeats steps 6 through 8 for two additional readings. Notes highest reading of three as patient's PEFR.		
10.	Disinfects equipment and discards supplies.		
11.	Removes and discards gloves. Washes hands.		
12.	Documents procedure using facility guidelines.		

Date Reviewed ____________ Instructor Signature ____________

Date Performed ____________ Instructor Signature ____________

Name: ______________________

Obtaining a throat culture

	Procedure Steps	yes	no
1.	Identifies self by name. Identifies patient.		
2.	Washes hands.		
3.	Explains procedure to patient, speaking clearly, slowly, and directly. Maintains face-to-face contact whenever possible.		
4.	Gathers required equipment.		
5.	Puts on gloves and other PPE as required.		
6.	Removes swab from its packaging.		
7.	Asks patient to tilt head back slightly, open mouth, and say "Ahhhh."		
8.	Uses tongue depressor to hold tongue down. Inserts swab in patient's mouth. Rubs it along tonsils and back of throat, avoiding uvula.		
9.	Removes swab and tongue depressor. Allows patient to close mouth.		
10.	Places swab in its transport vial/ tube.		
11.	Labels tube in front of patient, initialing and noting time and date of swab. Confirms identifying information on label. Prepares sealed tube and paperwork for transport. Properly discards all waste.		
12.	Removes and discards gloves. Washes hands.		
13.	Documents procedure using facility guidelines.		

Date Reviewed ____________ Instructor Signature ____________

Date Performed ____________ Instructor Signature ____________

Collecting a sputum specimen

	Procedure Steps	yes	no
1.	Identifies self by name. Identifies patient.		
2.	Washes hands.		
3.	Explains procedure to patient, speaking clearly, slowly, and directly. Maintains face-to-face contact whenever possible.		
4.	Puts on mask and gloves. Stands behind patient if patient can hold specimen container.		
5.	Asks patient to cough deeply. Gives patient tissues to cover mouth while coughing. Asks patient to spit sputum into container.		
6.	After sample has been obtained, covers container tightly and wipes any sputum off outside of container. Applies label with initials and time of collection. Places container in a clean specimen bag. Seals bag.		
7.	Removes and discards gloves and mask. Washes hands.		
8.	Takes specimen and lab slip to proper area.		
9.	Documents procedure using facility guidelines.		

Date Reviewed ____________ Instructor Signature ____________

Date Performed ____________ Instructor Signature ____________

Testing urine with reagent strips

	Procedure Steps	yes	no
1.	Washes hands.		
2.	Puts on gloves.		
3.	Confirms that strips are not expired.		

Name: ______________________

4.	Takes strip and recaps bottle, closing bottle tightly.		
5.	Dips strip into specimen.		
6.	Follows manufacturer's instructions for when to remove strip from specimen. Removes strip at correct time.		
7.	Waits appropriate time before comparing strip with color chart on bottle. Does not touch bottle with strip.		
8.	Reads results.		
9.	Stores strips. Discards used items. Discards specimen according to facility policy.		
10.	Removes and discards gloves. Washes hands.		
11.	Documents procedure using facility guidelines.		

Date Reviewed ______ Instructor Signature ______

Date Performed ______ Instructor Signature ______

Collecting a clean-catch (midstream) urine specimen

	Procedure Steps	yes	no
1.	Identifies self by name. Identifies patient.		
2.	Washes hands.		
3.	Explains procedure to patient, speaking clearly, slowly, and directly. Maintains face-to-face contact whenever possible.		
4.	Labels specimen container in front of patient. Initials it and notes time and date of collection. Asks patient to confirm identifying information on label.		
5.	Gives patient wipes required (2 for males; 3 for females). Instructs patient to collect specimen properly.		
6.	After patient provides specimen, MA puts on gloves.		
7.	Takes urine specimen from patient or retrieves it from drop location.		
8.	Prepares specimen and paperwork for transport.		
9.	Removes and discards gloves. Washes hands.		

Date Reviewed ______ Instructor Signature ______

Date Performed ______ Instructor Signature ______

Performing fecal occult blood testing

	Procedure Steps	yes	no
1.	Identifies self by name. Identifies patient.		
2.	Instructs patient to wash hands thoroughly before and after collecting or handling specimens.		
3.	Reviews instructions for preparation and collection.		
4.	Demonstrates how to collect specimen.		
5.	Instructs patient to label specimen according to facility guidelines. Describes how and when patient should return test.		
6.	To test a specimen, first washes hands. Puts on gloves. Removes card from specimen bag. Verifies that patient identification matches specimen label.		
7.	Opens flap on back of card.		
8.	Applies reagent to each square.		
9.	Reads results of test as instructed.		

10.	Discards testing card in a biohazardous waste container.		
11.	Removes and discards gloves. Washes hands.		
12.	Reports results to provider.		
13.	Documents procedure according to facility guidelines.		

Date Reviewed ______________ Instructor Signature ______________

Date Performed ______________ Instructor Signature ______________

Assisting with a pelvic exam and Pap test

	Procedure Steps	yes	no
1.	Identifies self by name. Identifies patient.		
2.	Washes hands.		
3.	Explains procedure to patient, speaking clearly, slowly, and directly. Maintains face-to-face contact whenever possible.		
4.	Gives patient gown and drape. Explains which clothing to remove and how to use gown and drape.		
5.	Gathers required equipment.		
6.	Washes hands. Puts on gloves and other PPE as required.		
7.	Warms speculum.		
8.	Applies lubricant to speculum.		
9.	Helps provider during examination as needed.		
10.	Places microscope slides within provider's reach.		
11.	Applies fixative immediately after provider collects cervical cell specimen.		
12.	Labels each slide with patient's identifying information. Notes site from which specimen is taken.		
13.	Allows slides to dry completely.		
14.	Places slides in a slide case and places slide case in a biohazardous specimen bag. Records date and time of collection on requisition.		
15.	Removes gloves and washes hands.		
16.	Helps patient to sit up. Provides tissues or wipes. Provides privacy for dressing.		
17.	Documents procedure using facility guidelines.		
18.	Follows facility policy for transporting specimens to lab.		

Date Reviewed ______________ Instructor Signature ______________

Date Performed ______________ Instructor Signature ______________

Performing allergy scratch testing

	Procedure Steps	yes	no
1.	Identifies self by name. Identifies patient.		
2.	Washes hands.		
3.	Explains procedure to patient, speaking clearly, slowly, and directly. Maintains face-to-face contact whenever possible.		
4.	Makes sure that patient has not taken restricted drugs during past 5–7 days.		
5.	Gives patient a gown. Asks patient to change into gown with opening in back. Provides privacy for changing.		
6.	Returns and helps patient to correct position (seated for forearm, prone for back).		
7.	Puts on gloves.		

Name: ______________________

8.	Cleans skin site for testing. Allows to dry.		
9.	Applies a small drop of allergen extract to test site. Applies a small drop of control solution at least 1 inch (3.8 cm) from allergen test site.		
10.	Obtains lancet or needle and assists provider to scratch skin beneath allergen.		
11.	Discards lancet or needle in a sharps container.		
12.	Identifies allergen that was used with tape or marker.		
13.	Repeats steps 8–12 for each allergen used in testing. Uses a new lancet for each site.		
14.	Allows allergens to remain on test site for 20 minutes. Monitors patient for signs of severe reaction.		
15.	After test time, wipes sites with alcohol prep pad. Leaves labels in place.		
16.	Assists provider to assess test sites.		
17.	Discards any disposable items.		
18.	Applies cold pack if needed.		
19.	Disinfects exam room and equipment.		
20.	Removes and discards gloves. Washes hands.		
21.	Documents procedure using facility guidelines.		

Date Reviewed ____________ Instructor Signature ____________

Date Performed ____________ Instructor Signature ____________

Performing routine venipuncture with multisample needle and evacuated tube(s)

	Procedure Steps	yes	no
1.	Identifies self by name. Identifies patient.		
2.	Explains procedure to patient, speaking clearly, slowly, and directly. Maintains face-to-face contact whenever possible.		
3.	Gathers required equipment.		
4.	Washes hands. Puts on gloves and other PPE as required.		
5.	Asks patient to extend arms for visual inspection. Chooses an arm based on appearance of veins and patient's input.		
6.	Applies tourniquet to selected arm, 3–4 inches above bend in elbow. Asks patient to make (but not pump) a fist.		
7.	With a gloved index finger, palpates arm to find an acceptable vein. If a good site is not found, removes tourniquet. Applies it to other arm.		
8.	When a suitable site is located, releases tourniquet. Cleans site thoroughly. Applies friction with antiseptic agent.		
9.	Allows alcohol to dry fully. Does not blow on, fan, or wipe skin to speed drying. Assembles the needle and holder.		
10.	Reapplies tourniquet.		
11.	Anchors vein properly.		
12.	In a single, fluid motion, inserts needle into skin to puncture selected vein at an angle of less than 30 degrees.		

Name: ______________________________

13.	Inserts first collection tube. Releases tourniquet as soon as blood flow begins. Allows tube to fill completely.		
14.	If more than one tube is needed, replaces first filled tube with next tube. Uses proper order of draw. Continues until all needed tubes are filled.		
15.	Places a piece of gauze, folded into quarters, over needle.		
16.	Removes needle from patient's arm. Engages safety device. Discards needle and holder in a sharps container. Keeps pressure on gauze, asking patient to help if able. Does not allow patient to bend arm up.		
17.	Mixes tubes appropriately.		
18.	Labels tubes in front of patient. Initials each one. Notes time and date of collection. Asks patient to check identifying information on label. Prepares specimens and paperwork for transport. Properly discards waste.		
19.	Checks that patient has stopped bleeding.		
20.	Places a bandage over gauze at puncture site. Tells patient to leave bandage in place for 15 minutes.		
21.	Observes patient for signs of dizziness or discomfort.		
22.	Removes and discards gloves. Washes hands.		
23.	Documents procedure using facility guidelines.		

Date Reviewed	Instructor Signature
Date Performed	Instructor Signature

Collecting a blood specimen using a syringe and transfer device

	Procedure Steps	yes	no
1.	Identifies self by name. Identifies patient.		
2.	Explains procedure to patient, speaking clearly, slowly, and directly. Maintains face-to-face contact whenever possible.		
3.	Gathers required equipment.		
4.	Washes hands. Puts on gloves and other PPE.		
5.	Asks patient to extend hands, palms down, for visual inspection. Chooses a hand based on appearance of veins. (If drawing from antecubital fossa, selects an appropriate vein.)		
6.	Applies tourniquet 3–4 inches above selected area. Asks patient to make (but not pump) a fist.		
7.	With a gloved index finger, palpates vein and chooses best site for puncture. If a good site is not found, removes tourniquet. Applies it to other side.		
8.	When a good site is found, releases tourniquet. Cleans and dries site properly.		
9.	Assembles needle and syringe.		
10.	Prepares syringe for use.		
11.	Reapplies tourniquet.		
12.	Anchors vein properly.		
13.	In a single, fluid motion, inserts needle into skin to puncture selected vein at the lowest possible angle.		
14.	Secures needle of a winged collection set throughout draw, following CLSI standards.		
15.	Pulls back gently and steadily on syringe plunger until needed amount of blood is drawn.		

16.	Places a piece of gauze, folded into quarters, over needle.		
17.	Removes needle from patient's arm. Engages safety device. Keeps pressure on gauze, asking patient to help if able.		
18.	Removes flexible tubing from syringe. Discards needle and tubing in a sharps container.		
19.	Immediately screws syringe onto syringe transfer device.		
20.	Inserts needed collection tube(s), following order of draw. Does not press on syringe plunger as blood transfers.		
21.	Discards syringe and transfer device in a sharps container.		
22.	Mixes tubes appropriately.		
23.	Labels tubes in front of patient. Initials each one. Notes time and date of collection. Asks patient to check identifying information on label. Prepares specimens and paperwork for transport. Properly discards waste.		
24.	Checks that patient has stopped bleeding.		
25.	Places a bandage over gauze at puncture site. Tells patient to leave bandage in place for 15 minutes.		
26.	Observes patient for signs of dizziness or discomfort.		
27.	Removes and discards gloves. Washes hands.		
28.	Documents procedure using facility guidelines.		

Date Reviewed ____________ Instructor Signature ____________

Date Performed ____________ Instructor Signature ____________

Performing routine capillary puncture

	Procedure Steps	yes	no
1.	Identifies self by name. Identifies patient.		
2.	Explains procedure to patient, speaking clearly, slowly, and directly. Maintains face-to-face contact whenever possible.		
3.	Gathers required equipment.		
4.	Washes hands. Puts on gloves and other PPE as required.		
5.	Asks patient to extend her hands, palms up, for visual inspection. Chooses a site free of bruising, rashes, broken skin, swelling, or cyanosis.		
6.	Warms site if required.		
7.	Cleans selected puncture site thoroughly, creating gentle friction. Allows site to dry fully.		
8.	Prepares lancet and collection devices for use.		
9.	Places lancet on patient's skin at selected site and activates it to puncture skin.		
10.	Discards used lancet in sharps container.		
11.	Uses gauze square to wipe away first drop of blood if required.		
12.	Collects patient's blood in required container(s). Applies gentle pressure. Does not squeeze or "milk" finger or heel. Gently applies and then releases pressure. Does not touch spout or any part of collection device to patient's skin. Gently taps collection tube as blood enters.		

13.	Continues to hold patient's finger or heel and collection device in place until container is filled to appropriate level. After filling, caps/seals specimens as instructed. Mixes them promptly (as needed).		
14.	After all needed containers are filled, places gauze over puncture site. Keeps pressure on gauze, asking patient to help if able.		
15.	Labels tubes in front of patient. Initials each one. Notes time and date of collection. Asks patient to check that identifying information on label is correct. Prepares specimens and paperwork for transport. Properly discards waste.		
16.	Checks that patient has stopped bleeding.		
17.	Places a bandage over puncture site if patient is over 2 years old. Tells patient to leave bandage in place for 15 minutes.		
18.	Observes patient for any signs of dizziness or discomfort.		
19.	Removes and discards gloves. Washes hands.		
20.	Documents procedure using facility guidelines.		

______ Date Reviewed ______ Instructor Signature

______ Date Performed ______ Instructor Signature

Obtaining a 12-lead EKG

	Procedure Steps	yes	no
1.	Identifies self by name. Identifies patient.		
2.	Washes hands.		
3.	Explains procedure to patient, speaking clearly, slowly, and directly. Maintains face-to-face contact whenever possible. Explains to male patient that chest hair may need to be clipped for proper electrode contact. Reassures patient that test is painless and takes only a few minutes.		
4.	Asks patient to undress from waist up and put gown on with opening facing forward. Follows facility procedures about asking patients to remove jewelry and about asking a female patient to remove or leave on her bra. Asks patient to remove socks or stockings that would prevent electrodes from being placed on lower extremities (unless placing LL and RL electrodes on torso). Provides privacy for patient to change.		
5.	After returning to room, puts on gloves.		
6.	Assists patient into supine position.		
7.	Places EKG machine beside bed and plugs it into an electrical outlet.		
8.	Turns machine on and waits until it completes self-tests.		
9.	Enters patient's information into machine. Ensures the machine is showing right patient information.		
10.	Prepares patient's skin, if needed, by drying or removing lotion or by clipping hair. Throughout procedure, exposes only areas necessary to prepare skin and run test.		
11.	Opens package of electrodes and attaches one electrode to each lead wire by snapping or clipping.		

Name: ______________________

12.	Attaches electrodes in correct positions, keeping patient covered as much as possible. Avoids bony areas, broken skin, scar tissue, and skin over implanted devices.		
13.	Asks patient to relax and be as still as possible.		
14.	When tracing is clear on monitor or when machine shows a green light, prints EKG according to manufacturer's instructions.		
15.	Checks EKG for evidence of lethal dysrhythmias or ST segment abnormalities. If any are seen, tells provider immediately.		
16.	Disconnects lead wires, taking care not to pull on patient's skin. Asks patient to remove and discard electrodes. If patient is not able to do this, removes electrodes gently and discards them.		
17.	Removes and discards gloves. Washes hands.		
18.	Tells patient where to place gown and gives them privacy for dressing.		
19.	Uploads or files EKG into patient's medical record. Documents procedure using facility guidelines.		
20.	Cleans and stores EKG machine and equipment.		
21.	Washes hands.		

Date Reviewed ______________ Instructor Signature ______________

Date Performed ______________ Instructor Signature ______________

Conducting an exercise stress test

	Procedure Steps	yes	no
1.	Identifies self by name. Identifies patient.		
2.	Washes hands.		
3.	Explains procedure to patient, speaking clearly, slowly, and directly. Maintains face-to-face contact whenever possible. Explains to male patient that chest hair may need to be clipped for proper electrode contact. Reassures patient that test is painless.		
4.	Correctly calculates target heart rate for stress test. Records in patient's chart.		
5.	Puts on gloves. Correctly obtains patient's baseline 12-lead EKG, placing limb electrodes on torso or near torso.		
6.	Assists patient to a seated position.		
7.	Applies sphygmomanometer cuff and pulse oximetry probe to patient.		
8.	Obtains and records baseline measurements for blood pressure, oxygen saturation, heart rate, and respirations. Sets monitor to read blood pressure as often as directed.		
9.	Tells provider when patient is ready to start test.		
10.	Repeats EKG every 2–3 minutes according to facility guidelines.		
11.	Monitors patient's EKG, heart rate, blood pressure, respirations, and oxygen saturation readings during test.		
12.	Assists provider as requested.		

13.	Continues to monitor patient when stress test is completed. Waits until EKG, heart rate, blood pressure, respirations, and oxygen saturation return to baseline.		
14.	Disconnects lead wires, taking care not to pull on patient's skin. Asks patient to remove and discard electrodes. If patient is not able to do this, removes electrodes gently and discards them.		
15.	Removes and discards gloves. Washes hands.		
16.	Gives patient privacy for dressing.		
17.	Uploads or files EKG and other data into patient's medical record. Documents procedure using facility guidelines.		
18.	Cleans and stores equipment.		
19.	Washes hands.		

Date Reviewed	Instructor Signature
Date Performed	Instructor Signature

Applying an ambulatory monitor

	Procedure Steps	yes	no
1.	Identifies self by name. Identifies patient.		
2.	Washes hands.		
3.	Explains procedure to patient, speaking clearly, slowly, and directly. Maintains face-to-face contact whenever possible. Explains to male patient that chest hair may need to be clipped for proper electrode contact. Reassures patient that test is painless.		
4.	Asks patient to undress from waist up and put gown on with opening facing forward. Follows facility procedures about asking patients to remove jewelry and about asking a female patient to remove or leave on her bra. Provides privacy for patient to change.		
5.	Puts on gloves.		
6.	Prepares patient's skin, if needed, by drying or removing lotion or by clipping hair that would stop electrodes from sticking. Throughout procedure, exposes only areas necessary to prepare skin and place electrodes.		
7.	Opens package of electrodes and attaches one electrode to each lead wire by snapping or clipping. Follows facility policy about use of stress loops.		
8.	Attaches electrodes in correct positions. Avoids bony areas, broken skin, scar tissue, and skin over implanted devices.		
9.	Removes and discards gloves. Washes hands.		
10.	Gives patient instructions for type of monitoring ordered, including directions for returning monitor. Allows patient to ask any questions he may have. Reinforces instructions.		
11.	Gives patient privacy for dressing.		
12.	Documents procedure using facility guidelines.		

Date Reviewed	Instructor Signature
Date Performed	Instructor Signature

Name: ______________________

Administering oral medications

	Procedure Steps	yes	no
1.	Identifies self by name. Identifies patient.		
2.	Washes hands.		
3.	Explains procedure to patient, speaking clearly, slowly, and directly. Maintains face-to-face contact whenever possible.		
4.	Puts on gloves if required.		
5.	Makes sure patient is in an upright sitting position.		
6.	Provides medication(s) to patient.		
7.	Observes as patient swallows medication.		
8.	Discards any disposable items or trash.		
9.	Removes and discards gloves if used. Washes hands.		
10.	Documents administration of medication(s) using facility guidelines.		

Date Reviewed ______ Instructor Signature ______

Date Performed ______ Instructor Signature ______

Administering buccal and sublingual medications

	Procedure Steps	yes	no
1.	Identifies self by name. Identifies patient.		
2.	Washes hands.		
3.	Explains procedure to patient, speaking clearly, slowly, and directly. Maintains face-to-face contact whenever possible.		
4.	Puts on gloves if required.		
5.	Makes sure patient is in an upright sitting position.		
6.	Provides medication to patient. For buccal route, tells patient to place medication between cheek and gums. For sublingual route, tells patient to place medication under his tongue. Helps as needed.		
7.	Tells patient to let medication dissolve in place without chewing or swallowing.		
8.	Does not leave room until medication has been placed and dissolved. Does not offer fluids until medication has dissolved completely.		
9.	Discards any disposable items or trash.		
10.	Removes and discards gloves if used. Washes hands.		
11.	Documents administration of medication(s) using facility guidelines.		

Date Reviewed ______ Instructor Signature ______

Date Performed ______ Instructor Signature ______

Administering medications by metered dose inhaler

	Procedure Steps	yes	no
1.	Identifies self by name. Identifies patient.		
2.	Washes hands.		
3.	Explains procedure to patient, speaking clearly, slowly, and directly. Maintains face-to-face contact whenever possible.		
4.	Makes sure patient is in an upright sitting position.		
5.	Puts on gloves if required.		
6.	Shakes inhaler vigorously for approximately 5 seconds.		

7.	Removes cap from mouthpiece. Checks mouthpiece for any foreign object or dust.		
	If spacer is used:		
8.	Inserts inhaler mouthpiece into spacer.		
9.	If patient uses a mask with spacer, places spacer mask over nose and mouth to form a tight seal. If not, asks patient to put spacer mouthpiece between teeth and form a seal around it. Holds inhaler properly. As needed, supports spacer with other hand, or asks patient to hold it.		
10.	Presses down firmly and quickly on canister to release medicine into spacer.		
11.	Encourages patient to breathe in slowly. If a whistle sounds, asks patient to slow breathing.		
	If spacer is not used:		
8.	Holds inhaler with a thumb underneath plastic case and index finger on top of medicine canister.		
9.	Tells patient inhaler will be activated on count of 3. Asks him to breathe in steadily when medication is released.		
10.	Instructs patient to breathe in and out. Places inhaler between his teeth. Asks him to seal his lips around mouthpiece.		
11.	Counts to 3, then presses down firmly and quickly on canister. Encourages patient to breathe in.		
	For both methods:		
12.	When medication has been inhaled, asks patient to hold his breath for 5 seconds (or as directed).		
13.	If more than 1 inhalation is ordered, waits approximately 1 minute before second inhalation. Shakes inhaler again before administering a second inhalation.		
14.	If medication is a corticosteroid, asks patient to rinse.		
15.	Replaces cap(s) on inhaler and spacer (if used).		
16.	Makes patient comfortable.		
17.	Cleans and stores reusable equipment. Discards trash.		
18.	Removes and discards gloves if used. Washes hands.		
19.	Reports any changes in patient to provider.		
20.	Documents administration of medication(s) using facility guidelines.		

Date Reviewed	Instructor Signature
Date Performed	Instructor Signature

Administering medications by nebulizer

	Procedure Steps	yes	no
1.	Identifies self by name. Identifies patient.		
2.	Washes hands.		
3.	Explains procedure to patient, speaking clearly, slowly, and directly. Maintains face-to-face contact whenever possible.		
4.	Puts on gloves if required.		
5.	Positions patient in an upright sitting position.		
6.	Removes lid from medication chamber. Empties ordered vials into chamber. Replaces lid on medication chamber.		

Name: ____________________

7.	Attaches tubing from nebulizer to medication chamber. Attaches ordered delivery device (mask, etc.) to medication chamber.		
8.	Places mask over patient's nose and mouth, or asks patient to place mouthpiece in mouth with lips closed around mouthpiece.		
9.	Turns nebulizer on. Encourages patient using a mask to breathe normally. Encourages patient using mouthpiece to breathe in through mouth and out through nose.		
10.	Continues nebulizer use until no medication remains or for ordered time.		
11.	After medication has been administered, assists patient to remove mask or mouthpiece.		
12.	Cleans and stores reusable equipment. Discards trash.		
13.	Removes and discards gloves if used. Washes hands.		
14.	Reports any changes in patient to provider.		
15.	Documents administration of medication(s) using facility guidelines.		

Date Reviewed ____________ Instructor Signature ____________

Date Performed ____________ Instructor Signature ____________

Administering nasal medications

	Procedure Steps	yes	no
1.	Identifies self by name. Identifies patient.		
2.	Washes hands.		
3.	Explains procedure to patient, speaking clearly, slowly, and directly. Maintains face-to-face contact whenever possible.		
4.	Puts on gloves if required.		
5.	Gives patient a tissue and asks her to blow her nose gently.		
6.	Positions patient properly. If administering a nasal spray, ensures patient is in an upright sitting position with head tilted slightly forward. For nasal drops, ensures patient is lying flat on her back.		
7.	Administers medication. For nasal spray, shakes medication, then places nozzle into one nostril and squeezes to administer. Places nozzle into other nostril and squeezes to administer. Repeats if multiple sprays are ordered. For nasal drops, does not touch dropper to outside of nose or nostril. Squeezes dropper and allows ordered number of drops to fall into patient's nostril, toward septum.		
8.	Asks patient to wait at least a minute before wiping or blowing her nose.		
9.	Cleans and stores reusable equipment. Discards any trash.		
10.	Removes and discards gloves. Washes hands.		
11.	Documents administration of medication(s) using facility guidelines.		

Date Reviewed ____________ Instructor Signature ____________

Date Performed ____________ Instructor Signature ____________

Name: ______________________________

Administering ophthalmic (eye) medications			
	Procedure Steps	yes	no
1.	Identifies self by name. Identifies patient.		
2.	Washes hands.		
3.	Explains procedure to patient, speaking clearly, slowly, and directly. Maintains face-to-face contact whenever possible.		
4.	Puts on gloves.		
5.	Uses a tissue to gently wipe patient's eye from inside corner (inner canthus) to outside. If medication will be administered to both eyes, uses a new tissue to wipe other eye.		
6.	Positions patient properly, with head tilted back.		
7.	Using a gloved finger, pulls lower eyelid down slightly, forming a pocket (gap) between lower lid and eye. Tells patient to look up.		
	For eye drops:		
8.	Fills medicine dropper or points tip of bottle downward if it has a built-in dropper. Instills a drop of medication into gap between lid and eye. Does not touch eye with dropper.		
9.	Asks patient to close eye. Presses gently on inner canthus for 1 minute. Repeats as needed. Waits 5 minutes before instilling a second drop as needed. Repeats with second eye if ordered.		
	For ointment:		
8.	Carefully squeezes a line of ointment into gap between eye and lower lid. Does not touch tip of tube to eyelid or eye. Repeats with second eye if ordered.		
9.	Asks patient to gently close eyes and leave them closed for several minutes.		
	For both forms:		
10.	Uses clean tissues to remove extra drops or ointment from around patient's eyes. Uses a new tissue for each eye.		
11.	Makes patient comfortable.		
12.	Cleans and stores reusable equipment. Discards any disposable items or trash.		
13.	Removes and discards gloves. Washes hands.		
14.	Documents administration of medication(s) using facility guidelines.		

__________ Date Reviewed   ______________ Instructor Signature

__________ Date Performed   ______________ Instructor Signature

Administering otic (ear) medications			
	Procedure Steps	yes	no
1.	Identifies self by name. Identifies patient.		
2.	Washes hands.		
3.	Explains procedure to patient, speaking clearly, slowly, and directly. Maintains face-to-face contact whenever possible.		
4.	Puts on gloves if required.		
5.	Positions patient properly.		
6.	Uses cotton ball to wipe away moisture or debris from outer ear.		

Name: ______________________

7.	Straightens ear canal. Gently pulls up and back on outside edge of ear (down and back for children under 3). Fills medicine dropper or points tip of bottle with built-in dropper downward. Instills ordered number of drops to ear. Allows liquid to run down side of ear canal.		
8.	Places a clean cotton ball over ear canal. (Does not insert it into ear canal.) Asks patient to stay in same position for 3–5 minutes. Repeats with second ear if ordered.		
9.	Helps patient to a comfortable position.		
10.	Cleans and stores reusable equipment. Discards any disposable items or trash.		
11.	Removes and discards gloves if used. Washes hands.		
12.	Documents administration of medication(s) using facility guidelines.		

Date Reviewed ______ Instructor Signature ______

Date Performed ______ Instructor Signature ______

Administering topical medications

	Procedure Steps	yes	no
1.	Identifies self by name. Identifies patient.		
2.	Washes hands.		
3.	Explains procedure to patient, speaking clearly, slowly, and directly. Maintains face-to-face contact whenever possible.		
4.	Puts on gloves if required.		
5.	Positions patient properly. Exposes only body part to which medication will be applied.		
6.	Follows medication order and manufacturer's instructions for application.		
7.	Discards used application devices.		
8.	Makes patient comfortable.		
9.	Cleans and stores reusable equipment. Discards trash.		
10.	Removes and discards gloves if used. Washes hands.		
11.	Documents administration of medication(s) using facility guidelines.		

Date Reviewed ______ Instructor Signature ______

Date Performed ______ Instructor Signature ______

Administering transdermal (patch) medications

	Procedure Steps	yes	no
1.	Identifies self by name. Identifies patient.		
2.	Washes hands.		
3.	Explains procedure to patient, speaking clearly, slowly, and directly. Maintains face-to-face contact whenever possible.		
4.	Puts on gloves if required.		
5.	Positions patient properly. Exposes only body part to which medication patch will be applied.		
6.	If a patch is already in place, removes it. Cleans site as directed.		
7.	Does not touch patch with bare hands. Discards it so that no other person may accidentally touch it.		
8.	Removes and discards gloves. Washes hands and puts on new gloves.		

9.	Writes initials, date, and time on patch if required.		
10.	Applies new transdermal patch properly.		
11.	Removes and discards gloves. Washes hands.		
12.	Makes patient comfortable.		
13.	Documents administration of medication(s) using facility guidelines.		

Date Reviewed ____________ Instructor Signature ____________

Date Performed ____________ Instructor Signature ____________

Administering a rectal suppository

	Procedure Steps	yes	no
1.	Identifies self by name. Identifies patient.		
2.	Washes hands.		
3.	Explains procedure to patient speaking clearly, slowly, and directly. Maintains face-to-face contact whenever possible.		
4.	Asks patient to remove clothing from waist down. Gives patient drape and leaves room for privacy.		
5.	Helps patient into Sims' position. Covers with drape.		
6.	Uncovers patient enough to expose buttocks only.		
7.	Unwraps suppository.		
8.	Puts on gloves.		
9.	Lubricates suppository as needed.		
10.	Spreads buttocks to expose anal area.		
11.	Using index finger, inserts suppository. Places suppository past rectal sphincter against wall of colon.		
12.	Asks patient to take deep breaths and retain suppository.		
13.	Withdraws finger and briefly holds toilet paper against anus. Discards toilet paper.		
14.	Discards trash.		
15.	Removes and discards gloves. Washes hands.		
16.	Tells patient where to place drape and gives him privacy for dressing.		
17.	Documents administration of medication(s) using facility guidelines.		

Date Reviewed ____________ Instructor Signature ____________

Date Performed ____________ Instructor Signature ____________

Administering medications by the vaginal route

	Procedure Steps	yes	no
1.	Identifies self by name. Identifies patient.		
2.	Washes hands.		
3.	Explains procedure to patient, speaking clearly, slowly, and directly. Maintains face-to-face contact whenever possible.		
4.	Asks patient to remove clothing from waist down. Gives patient a drape and leaves room for privacy.		
5.	Helps patient into dorsal recumbent position and covers her with drape.		
6.	Unwraps suppository or prepares medication applicator. If using an applicator, inspects it for breaks, cracks, or rough edges.		
7.	Puts on gloves.		
8.	Lubricates suppository or applicator as needed.		

Name: ____________________

9.	Inserts suppository or applicator into vagina 2–3 inches. If using an applicator, presses plunger in fully to release medication, then removes and discards applicator. Does not force applicator into vagina if there is resistance.		
10.	Gently wipes area around vagina with a tissue if needed. Discards tissue.		
11.	Removes and discards gloves. Washes hands.		
12.	Tells patient where to place drape and gives her privacy for dressing.		
13.	Documents administration of medication(s) using facility guidelines.		

________________ Date Reviewed ________________ Instructor Signature

________________ Date Performed ________________ Instructor Signature

Reconstituting a powdered medication

	Procedure Steps	yes	no
1.	Washes hands.		
2.	Obtains medication vial. Checks medication label on vial against provider's order. Checks expiration dates of both vials. Discards expired vials.		
3.	Checks for right diluent. Notes amount of diluent needed.		
4.	Removes caps from diluent and medication vials. Cleans rubber tops.		
5.	Places vials upright on work surface. Prepares a hypodermic needle and syringe.		
6.	Checks medication label against provider's order again. Checks amount of diluent again.		
7.	Removes needle cap and inserts hypodermic needle into medication vial. Does not touch powdered medication with needle. Pulls syringe back to remove amount of air that will be replaced with diluent.		
8.	Removes needle from medication vial. Places vial on work surface and cleans rubber top with an alcohol prep pad.		
9.	Inserts needle into diluent vial. Keeps needle's bevel below level of fluid.		
10.	Holds vial between middle and index fingers of nondominant hand and turns it upside down. Uses other fingers and thumb to secure syringe.		
11.	Pushes in plunger of syringe completely to inject all air into diluent vial. Withdraws correct amount of diluent from vial. Adjusts position of needle as needed to keep it below level of liquid in vial.		
12.	Gently taps barrel of syringe to move air bubbles to top.		
13.	Carefully pushes plunger to remove air bubbles. Checks that proper dose of diluent is in syringe.		
14.	Removes needle from vial.		
15.	Checks label on medication vial against provider's order again.		
16.	Inserts needle and syringe containing diluent into medication vial.		
17.	Pushes in plunger of syringe completely to inject all of diluent into medication vial.		

18.	Removes needle from medication vial. Activates safety device. Discards needle and syringe in sharps container.		
19.	Mixes medication carefully by rolling it between palms. Places vial upright on work surface.		
20.	Discards waste and cleans work surface.		

Date Reviewed ____ Instructor Signature ____

Date Performed ____ Instructor Signature ____

Preparing injection medications in vials

	Procedure Steps	yes	no
1.	Washes hands.		
2.	Obtains medication vial. Checks medication label on vial against provider's order. Checks expiration date. Discards expired vials.		
3.	Removes cap (if still intact) from vial. Cleans rubber top with an alcohol prep pad.		
4.	Mixes medication carefully by rolling it between palms. Places vial upright on work surface.		
5.	Opens syringe. Attaches a needle for drawing up medication if one is not already attached. Pulls plunger of syringe back to correct marking for medication dose.		
6.	Removes needle cap. Inserts needle into vial. Keeps bevel below level of fluid.		
7.	Holds vial between middle and index fingers of nondominant hand and turns it upside down. Uses remaining fingers and thumb to secure syringe.		
8.	Pushes in plunger of syringe completely to inject all air into vial.		
9.	Gently pulls back on syringe to withdraw correct dose of medication from vial. Adjusts position of needle as needed to keep it below level of liquid in vial.		
10.	Removes needle from vial.		
11.	Gently taps barrel of syringe to move any air bubbles to top.		
12.	Carefully pushes plunger to remove air bubbles. Confirms that proper dose of medication has been withdrawn.		
13.	Removes needle. Discards it in sharps container.		
14.	Checks medication label against provider's order again.		
15.	If vial is glass and held a single dose of medication, discards it in sharps container.		
16.	Attaches a new hypodermic needle to syringe.		
17.	Verifies medication and dose once more with provider's order. Labels syringe with name of medication and dose.		
18.	Discards waste and cleans work surface.		

Date Reviewed ____ Instructor Signature ____

Date Performed ____ Instructor Signature ____

Administering intradermal medications

	Procedure Steps	yes	no
1.	Draws up medication properly, checking order before and after drawing it up and before administering it.		
2.	Identifies self by name. Identifies patient.		
3.	Washes hands.		

Name: ____________________

4.	Explains procedure to patient, speaking clearly, slowly, and directly. Maintains face-to-face contact whenever possible.		
5.	Puts on gloves.		
6.	Chooses injection site. Chooses a site that is free from swelling, bruising, or scarring.		
7.	Cleans injection site with an alcohol prep pad. Allows it to dry.		
8.	Uses dominant hand to obtain medication syringe. Removes needle cap.		
9.	Pulls skin taut with nondominant hand. Holds syringe at a 10-degree angle to patient's skin.		
10.	With bevel up, inserts needle until bevel is beneath skin.		
11.	Uses nondominant hand to slowly push in syringe plunger and inject medication.		
12.	Removes needle from patient's skin. Activates safety device. Discards needle and syringe in sharps container.		
13.	Applies loose adhesive bandage if there is any bleeding.		
14.	Makes patient comfortable.		
15.	Discards trash.		
16.	Removes and discards gloves. Washes hands.		
17.	Documents administration of medication(s) using facility guidelines, including name of medication, dose administered, and location of injection.		

Date Reviewed ____________ Instructor Signature ____________

Date Performed ____________ Instructor Signature ____________

Administering subcutaneous medications			
	Procedure Steps	yes	no
1.	Draws up medication properly, checking order before and after drawing it up and before administering it.		
2.	Identifies self by name. Identifies patient.		
3.	Washes hands.		
4.	Explains procedure to patient, speaking clearly, slowly, and directly. Maintains face-to-face contact whenever possible.		
5.	Puts on gloves.		
6.	Chooses injection site. Chooses a site that is free from swelling, bruising, or scarring.		
7.	Cleans injection site with an alcohol prep pad. Allows it to dry.		
8.	Uses dominant hand to obtain medication syringe. Removes needle cap.		
9.	Using nondominant hand, pinches skin on each side of injection site.		
10.	Holds syringe at a 45-degree angle (or at 90-degree angle if patient has large amount of subcutaneous tissue).		
11.	With bevel up, inserts needle through skin until whole needle is inserted.		
12.	Pushes in syringe plunger slowly to inject medication.		
13.	Removes needle from patient's skin. Activates safety device. Covers injection site with gauze.		
14.	Discards needle and syringe in sharps container.		
15.	Applies adhesive bandage to injection site.		

16.	Makes patient comfortable.		
17.	Discards any trash.		
18.	Removes and discards gloves. Washes hands.		
19.	Documents administration of medication(s) using facility guidelines, including name of medication, dose administered, and location of injection.		

Date Reviewed ______ Instructor Signature ______

Date Performed ______ Instructor Signature ______

Administering intramuscular medications

	Procedure Steps	yes	no
1.	Draws up medication properly, checking order before and after drawing it up and before administering it.		
2.	Identifies self by name. Identifies patient.		
3.	Washes hands.		
4.	Explains procedure to patient, speaking clearly, slowly, and directly. Maintains face-to-face contact whenever possible.		
5.	Puts on gloves.		
6.	Chooses injection site. Chooses a site that is free from swelling, bruising, or scarring.		
7.	Cleans injection site with an alcohol prep pad. Allows it to dry.		
8.	Uses dominant hand to obtain medication syringe. Removes needle cap.		
9.	Using nondominant hand, holds skin at injection site taut. Holds syringe at a 90-degree angle to skin.		
10.	Inserts needle through skin until whole needle is inserted.		
11.	Pushes in syringe plunger slowly to inject medication.		
12.	Removes needle from patient's body. Activates safety device. Covers injection site with gauze.		
13.	Discards needle and syringe in sharps container.		
14.	Applies adhesive bandage to injection site.		
15.	Makes patient comfortable.		
16.	Discards any disposable items or trash.		
17.	Removes and discards gloves. Washes hands.		
18.	Documents administration of medication(s) using facility guidelines, including name of medication, dose administered, and location of injection.		

Date Reviewed ______ Instructor Signature ______

Date Performed ______ Instructor Signature ______

Name: ______________________________

Name: ______________________

Practice Exam

Multiple Choice

1. Which of the following is an example of an MA respecting patient confidentiality?
   (A) Not discussing details of the patient's care in the waiting room
   (B) Reviewing all medications with a patient during intake
   (C) Asking a patient to make a payment at the time of service
   (D) Initialing and dating any entries in a paper medical record

2. When a patient is providing a clean-catch (midstream) urine specimen, she must
   (A) Completely empty the bladder, then wait approximately 30 minutes and urinate again to provide the specimen
   (B) Save all urine produced over a 24-hour period
   (C) Provide the specimen in a bathroom where the water is turned off and dye is placed in the toilet
   (D) Clean the genital area properly, urinate a small amount into the toilet, and then urinate into the specimen container

3. What type of jewelry/accessory should be worn by an MA?
   (A) Any jewelry the MA wishes to wear
   (B) Earrings that dangle no more than ½ inch
   (C) A simple watch that can count seconds
   (D) An analog (not digital) watch with a second hand

4. What does the abbreviation *TPR* stand for?
   (A) Time, p-wave, and rhythm
   (B) Temperature, pulse, and respirations
   (C) Triglycerides, peptides, and renal function
   (D) Total parenteral respiration

5. What method may be used to add a suture packet to a sterile field?
   (A) The toss method
   (B) The drop method
   (C) The glove method
   (D) The mechanical method

6. A patient who takes an anxiolytic medication is likely to have a diagnosis of
   (A) Hypertension
   (B) Coronary artery disease
   (C) Generalized anxiety disorder
   (D) Osteoporosis

7. Which of the following is part of patient intake?
   (A) Providing the patient with a visit summary
   (B) Asking the patient what over-the-counter drugs and supplements they take
   (C) Drawing a blood specimen
   (D) Assessing the patient to give the doctor an idea of possible diagnoses

8. What are the male and female gametes?
   (A) Sperm and ova
   (B) Testosterone and estrogen
   (C) Testicles and ovaries
   (D) Penis and vagina

9. Using Standard Precautions includes
   (A) Always wearing gloves when providing patient care
   (B) Maintaining at least a 6-foot distance from patients
   (C) Limiting the number of patients sitting together in the waiting room
   (D) Wearing a gown and a mask/goggles or face shield when splashing or spraying of body fluids is likely

Name: ______________________________

10. In legal terms, a provider who sees another provider's patients on a temporary basis is a(n)
    (A) *Locum tenens*
    (B) Certified replacement provider
    (C) Designated physician
    (D) Arbiter

11. Which of the following laws relates to a patient's wishes about organ donation?
    (A) The Patient Self-Determination Act
    (B) The Health Insurance Portability and Accountability Act
    (C) The Uniform Anatomical Gift Act
    (D) The Genetic Information Nondiscrimination Act

12. The term *hematopoiesis* refers to
    (A) The production of insulin
    (B) The hardening of cartilage into bone
    (C) The creation of sex cells
    (D) The production of blood cells

13. A patient who recently had a left-sided mastectomy has an order for a complete blood count and a lipid panel. Which of the following is an acceptable site for collecting the specimen?
    (A) The middle or ring finger of either hand
    (B) The dorsal aspect of the right hand
    (C) The middle or ring finger of the right hand
    (D) The antecubital fossa of the right arm

14. An MA sends a patient this message through the patient portal: "Doc wants you to have a colonoscopy. Lucky you! Give us a call for prep instructions." What aspect of professionalism is missing from this message?
    (A) Empathy
    (B) Honesty
    (C) Dependability
    (D) Dedication

15. After drawing blood from one patient, an MA is asked to administer a flu shot to another patient. What must the MA do first?
    (A) Centrifuge the blood specimens
    (B) Wash his hands
    (C) Assess the second patient to see if a flu shot is needed
    (D) Document the flu shot in the second patient's record

16. Which of the following is an example of an autoimmune disease?
    (A) Osteoarthritis
    (B) Parkinson's disease
    (C) Rheumatoid arthritis
    (D) Gastroesophageal reflux disease

17. A patient's insurance requires payment of 10% of laboratory fees. This type of payment is called
    (A) A copayment
    (B) A premium
    (C) Coinsurance
    (D) A benefit

18. To determine the reorder point for an office or medical supply, the MA should
    (A) Multiply the amount of the item used each day by the number of days needed to get new supplies, then add the safety stock
    (B) Multiply the safety stock by the amount of the item used each day, then add the number of days needed to get new supplies
    (C) Add the safety stock to the number of days to get new supplies, then divide by the amount of the item used each day
    (D) Add together the amount of the item used each day, the number of days needed to get new supplies, and the safety stock

19. When placing electrodes for an EKG, the MA notes that the patient's body hair is keeping the electrodes from sticking well. If the MA does not correct the situation, which form of artifact is likely to appear?
    (A) Somatic tremor
    (B) Electrical interference
    (C) Broken recording
    (D) Wandering baseline

20. Before a patient has a needle biopsy performed in the medical office, the MA must be sure this is in the patient's record:
    (A) Results from any previous biopsies
    (B) A signed informed consent document
    (C) A signed general consent to treatment document
    (D) A referral from an oncologist

Name: ______________________________

21. When opening a medical office the MA should be sure that
    (A) The alarm is turned on
    (B) The provider has a list of all patients for the day and their anticipated diagnoses
    (C) The waiting room is clean and tidy
    (D) All patient files for the day are pulled and placed on the reception desk

22. An infant is receiving a DTaP vaccine, which is an intramuscular injection. Where will the vaccine be administered?
    (A) In the deltoid
    (B) In the ventrogluteal region
    (C) In the *vastus lateralis*
    (D) In the *gluteus maximus*

23. Which of the following is true of EKG leads?
    (A) They are circular, adhesive pads placed on a patient's body.
    (B) All forms of EKG testing use the same number of leads.
    (C) Each provides a different "view" of the heart's mechanical activity.
    (D) Each provides a different "view" of the heart's electrical activity.

24. This is generally part of patient intake at every visit for children and adults:
    (A) Measuring weight
    (B) Measuring head circumference
    (C) Measuring girth
    (D) Measuring height

25. Before a medical office sends an overdue account to collection, the MA may be asked to
    (A) Delete the patient's records
    (B) Call or send a letter to the patient to discuss payment options
    (C) Write a letter warning other providers that the patient has a poor payment record
    (D) Adjust the patient's account to reflect a zero balance

26. What should an MA do before placing a used venipuncture needle in a sharps container?
    (A) Recap the needle
    (B) Remove the needle from the tube holder
    (C) Activate the safety device
    (D) Bend the needle with forceps

27. Where in the body is a nasopharyngeal swab inserted?
    (A) In the ear
    (B) In the nostril
    (C) In the mouth
    (D) In the rectum

28. An MA accidentally injures a patient during routine, assigned care. What legal concept means the patient may sue the provider for damages?
    (A) *Res ipsa loquitur*
    (B) *Subpoena ad testificandum*
    (C) *Subpoena duces tecum*
    (D) *Respondeat superior*

29. Which of the following government-funded insurance programs is administered at the state level, with enrollment qualifications varying by state?
    (A) CHIP
    (B) TRICARE
    (C) IHS
    (D) CHAMPVA

30. A provider prescribes a new and expensive medication for a patient. What process will the MA likely have to manage to help the patient get the drug?
    (A) Preauthorization
    (B) Referral
    (C) Confirmation of benefits
    (D) Confirmation of diagnosis

31. This type of fracture is common in young children due to the immaturity of their bones:
    (A) Transverse fracture
    (B) Comminuted fracture
    (C) Greenstick fracture
    (D) Longitudinal fracture

32. How must paper documents that contain PHI be discarded?
    (A) They must be placed in two trash bags (double-bagged).
    (B) They must be shredded in such a way that the pieces cannot be put back together.
    (C) They must be shredded and then burned.
    (D) They must be stamped "CONFIDENTIAL" and then shredded.

Name: ______________________

33. When preparing a sterile field the MA should consider the outer ____ inch(es) to be nonsterile.
    (A) ½
    (B) 1
    (C) 2
    (D) 3

34. Which of the following is acceptable under HIPAA?
    (A) An MA talks to friends about patients if the friends will never meet the patient.
    (B) An MA talks about the care of a 19-year-old patient with the patient's mother, with whom she lives.
    (C) An MA talks to the provider about a patient while in the provider's private office.
    (D) An MA talks to the provider about a patient while in the waiting room.

35. A sign-in sheet often includes a field for the patient's
    (A) Phone number
    (B) Diagnosis
    (C) Appointment time
    (D) Medical record number

36. Where does the electrical impulse that triggers a heartbeat begin in a patient with a normal heart rhythm?
    (A) In the atrioventricular junction
    (B) In the Purkinje fibers
    (C) In the bundle of His
    (D) In the sinoatrial node

37. Which of the following collection tubes would be used first during venipuncture?
    (A) Lavender
    (B) Green
    (C) Gray
    (D) Light blue

38. Which of these items is part of the equipment a patient will need for a 24-hour urine specimen collection?
    (A) A 40-mL specimen container
    (B) A "hat" and/or a urinal
    (C) Tongue blades
    (D) A card with windows for placing drops of urine from different collection times

39. A hematologist sees patients with blood cancers on a certain day of the week. This is an example of
    (A) Wave scheduling
    (B) Open scheduling
    (C) Cluster scheduling
    (D) Timed scheduling

40. After a toddler receives routine vaccinations the provider orders a dose of acetaminophen to be administered before the patient leaves the office. The toddler weighs 32 pounds. The dosage for this weight is 160 mg. How many 80-mg chewable tablets should the MA administer?
    (A) ½
    (B) 1
    (C) 2
    (D) 3

41. This is an example of a salutation in a business letter:
    (A) Dear Mr. Qian:
    (B) RE: Test results
    (C) Yours sincerely, Alfredo Gonzales, MD
    (D) enc: Account statement

42. A medication is ordered for the treatment of conjunctivitis. Which of the following is true?
    (A) The MA must wear a mask and goggles while administering the drug.
    (B) The MA must wear gloves while administering the drug.
    (C) The patient must wear a mask while the drug is administered.
    (D) The MA must wear a gown while administering the drug.

43. An MA is performing a 12-lead EKG and sees that the ST segment is elevated. This could mean
    (A) That the patient is nervous
    (B) That the patient has a dysrhythmia that begins in the ventricles
    (C) That the patient is having a myocardial infarction
    (D) That the patient is having a stroke

Name: ______________________

44. An MA's best friend recently started dating a patient at the MA's office. The MA knows information about the patient's medical history that she thinks could affect her friend. Telling her friend this information is
    (A) Legal and ethical if not having the information could harm the friend
    (B) Legal but unethical
    (C) Legal and ethical if the patient tells the MA the information can be shared
    (D) Illegal and unethical

45. Which of the following is a surgical tool used for grasping and/or clamping?
    (A) Hemostat
    (B) Scalpel
    (C) Retractors
    (D) Biopsy punch

46. A patient whose thoracic spine has an abnormal posterior curvature has
    (A) Thoracic scoliosis
    (B) Lumbar scoliosis
    (C) Kyphosis
    (D) Lordosis

47. What ratio of bleach to water should be used to clean exam room surfaces?
    (A) 1:2
    (B) 1:5
    (C) 1:10
    (D) 1:15

48. Specimens for CLIA-waived PT/INR testing are collected by
    (A) Nasopharyngeal swab
    (B) Clean-catch (midstream) urine collection
    (C) Venipuncture
    (D) Capillary puncture

49. In an outpatient setting, which set of codes is most commonly used to bill for care provided during a patient visit?
    (A) ICD
    (B) CPT
    (C) HCPCS
    (D) HIPAA

50. Which of the following is true about patient consent?
    (A) Once a patient has signed a general consent form, no further consent is ever needed.
    (B) A patient who has signed a general consent form must sign a new form any time a routine test (e.g., venipuncture) is performed.
    (C) A patient who has signed a general consent form should still be asked for verbal consent before a routine test (e.g., venipuncture) is performed.
    (D) Consent is only needed for care that involves a risk of injury.

51. Wearing a high-quality respirator or mask (e.g., N95) may be required when caring for patients who have this type of illness:
    (A) Airborne
    (B) Contact-spread
    (C) Autoimmune
    (D) Bloodborne

52. At patient check-in, it is common to request
    (A) Payment for the day's visit
    (B) That the patient set up their next appointment
    (C) That the patient list the reason for their visit on a sign-in sheet
    (D) A urine specimen

53. An MA is setting up a sterile field for laceration repair. The date is 8/31/2024. The sterilization date for the laceration tray is 5/25/2024. Can this tray be used?
    (A) Yes
    (B) Only with authorization by the provider
    (C) Only if all instruments still appear clean
    (D) No

54. During one form of allergy testing the allergen is injected
    (A) Into the muscle tissue
    (B) Into the subcutaneous tissue
    (C) Just under the skin
    (D) Into a vein

Name: ______________________________

55. When should a bandage be applied to a venipuncture site?
    (A) Immediately after the needle is removed
    (B) After the patient has held gauze on the puncture site for 10 seconds
    (C) After the bleeding has slowed
    (D) After the bleeding has stopped
56. What type of testing is recommended every 5 years for female patients between 30 and 65 years old?
    (A) HPV testing
    (B) Pap testing
    (C) Co-testing (HPV and Pap testing together)
    (D) Bone density testing
57. How often do patients need to sign a medical office's privacy and consent documents?
    (A) Once a year
    (B) Only when the patient is first seen at an office
    (C) With every visit
    (D) Only when any information changes significantly
58. Which of the following must be reported to the CDC within 4 hours?
    (A) COVID-19
    (B) Botulism
    (C) Measles
    (D) Influenza
59. How might an MA help a patient who wants to stop smoking?
    (A) By sending encouraging messages through the patient portal
    (B) By providing a list of smoking cessation programs
    (C) By suggesting a nicotine patch
    (D) By sharing stories of patients who have lung cancer
60. After puncturing a patient's skin to collect a venipuncture specimen, the MA finds that blood will not flow. What should he do next?
    (A) Remove the tourniquet and the needle
    (B) Probe in all directions until blood flow is established
    (C) Gently adjust the needle slightly backward and forward
    (D) Call in the provider to assist
61. An EKG is ordered for a pediatric patient. The child is terrified and does not want to lie down for the test. Which of the following is the best response by the MA?
    (A) "Just this morning I did an EKG on a 2-year-old and he didn't cry. Can't you be brave like him?"
    (B) "We have lollipops for everyone who is brave during an EKG. Don't you want one?"
    (C) "I'm sorry you're scared, but if you can't get control of yourself I'll have to call in my friend to hold you down."
    (D) "I know this can be scary, but I promise it won't hurt. Do you want to hold one of these stickers that I'll put on you and see what it's like?"
62. When removing sutures, an MA should
    (A) Move from one end of the incision to the other
    (B) Start in the center and work out
    (C) Work inward from both ends of the incision
    (D) Try to clip two sutures at a time
63. A patient in a state where recreational marijuana use is legal reports during intake that they use marijuana about twice a month. What else should the MA ask?
    (A) What form and strength the patient uses
    (B) Whether anything the provider says could convince the patient to stop
    (C) Why the patient is making a choice that could harm their health
    (D) No other questions; frequency is the only needed information
64. A patient who weighs 65 kilograms asks the MA what her weight is in pounds. What is the correct answer?
    (A) 125 pounds
    (B) 137 pounds
    (C) 143 pounds
    (D) 151 pounds

65. As an MA is showing an elderly patient to an exam room, the patient stumbles and falls. The patient gets up on her own and says she is fine other than being embarrassed. What should the MA do?
   (A) Pretend the fall did not occur to protect the patient's dignity
   (B) Document the fall in the patient's medical record
   (C) Document the fall using the office's incident report form
   (D) Report the fall to OSHA

66. How is a patient typically positioned for a colonoscopy?
   (A) Supine position
   (B) Sims' position
   (C) Fowler's position
   (D) Dorsal recumbent position

67. During intake, a patient with asthma reports, "I've been mostly in green. I was yellow once last week." What is the patient likely referring to?
   (A) Peak expiratory flow rate measurements
   (B) Inhaler use
   (C) Perceived exertion levels
   (D) Home blood test results

68. During a lumbar puncture, fluid is removed from
   (A) The lungs
   (B) The bladder
   (C) A cyst
   (D) The subarachnoid space between vertebrae

69. Patients who are coughing in the waiting room should be
   (A) Asked to leave
   (B) Given a mask
   (C) Roomed immediately
   (D) Ignored

70. An MA sees that a patient's lab results have come back and that the patient's fasting blood glucose level was 203 mg/dL. The result is marked *HIGH*. What should the MA do?
   (A) Send the patient the office's diabetic diet guidelines through the patient portal
   (B) Call the patient and tell her she may have diabetes
   (C) Ensure that the provider sees the result
   (D) Tell the provider that the patient has diabetes

71. What must a patient who pays on a sliding scale provide to a medical office?
   (A) Verification of income
   (B) Proof of insurance
   (C) A bank statement
   (D) The name of a backup guarantor

72. Which of the following is part of providing weight-inclusive care?
   (A) Not weighing a patient at every visit
   (B) Making sure seating is available for patients of all sizes
   (C) Not using BMI as a screening tool
   (D) Discussing weight only if the patient mentions it

73. When sterilizing hinged instruments, the MA should place them
   (A) In a closed position
   (B) In an open position
   (C) Stacked together
   (D) Beneath an inverted (upside-down) bowl

74. When communicating with a patient who has a mental health disorder an MA should
   (A) Sit or stand slightly farther away from the patient than usual
   (B) Sit or stand directly beside the patient
   (C) Sit or stand at a normal distance from the patient
   (D) Sit or stand slightly closer to the patient than usual

Name: ______________________

75. What is the region of the brain where thinking, analysis, association of ideas, judgment, emotions, and memories occur?
    (A) The diencephalon
    (B) The cerebellum
    (C) The brain stem
    (D) The cerebral cortex

76. If an elderly patient comes to an appointment with his son, how is it best for the MA to communicate?
    (A) The MA should address only the son.
    (B) The MA should address only the patient.
    (C) The MA should ask that the provider manage all communication.
    (D) The MA should address the patient but should answer any questions from the son (within scope of practice).

77. A patient calls the medical office and says he believes he may be having a heart attack. How should the MA respond?
    (A) By putting the caller through to the provider immediately
    (B) By telling the caller to have someone take him to an urgent care center or emergency room immediately
    (C) By telling the caller to call or have someone else call 911 immediately
    (D) By coaching the caller through first aid for a heart attack

78. Using a code for a service that is less complicated than the service a provider performed will result in
    (A) The provider being overpaid
    (B) The provider being underpaid
    (C) The provider being audited
    (D) The patient receiving additional bills

79. Which of the following is a common antiseptic used when preparing for a blood culture?
    (A) Chlorhexidine gluconate
    (B) 60% isopropyl alcohol
    (C) Hydrogen peroxide
    (D) Mercurochrome

80. A wide QRS complex on an EKG tracing may indicate
    (A) Atrial fibrillation
    (B) Atherosclerosis
    (C) A ventricular dysrhythmia
    (D) An atrial dysrhythmia

81. When documenting in a patient's EHR on a computer that others can access, an MA must be sure to do this before walking away:
    (A) Close the patient's record and log out of their account on the program
    (B) Shut down the computer
    (C) Minimize all windows
    (D) Close the EHR program

82. A 60-year-old female patient reports that she has been experiencing urinary incontinence. What is the best follow-up question or statement by the MA?
    (A) "At your age, this is definitely to be expected."
    (B) "How often would you say this happens?"
    (C) "Have you tried limiting the amount of liquids you drink?"
    (D) "I'm sorry. That must be embarrassing."

83. Where could an MA refer a patient who is newly self-employed and looking for health insurance?
    (A) Medicare: medicare.gov
    (B) Medicaid: medicaid.gov
    (C) The Centers for Disease Control and Prevention: cdc.gov
    (D) Health insurance marketplace: healthcare.gov

84. During intake a patient suddenly has difficulty speaking and one side of her face is drooping. What may be happening to the patient?
    (A) She may be having a heart attack.
    (B) She may be having a stroke.
    (C) She may be having a tension headache.
    (D) She may be experiencing hypotension.

Name: ______________________________

85. A patient whose blood pressure is usually around 125/70 falls into this category:
(A) Normal blood pressure
(B) Elevated blood pressure
(C) Stage 1 hypertension
(D) Stage 2 hypertension

86. Which of the following should an MA tell a patient not to do while wearing an ambulatory heart monitor?
(A) Have sexual intercourse
(B) Eat heavy meals
(C) Swim
(D) Run

87. Lisinopril, amlodipine, and metoprolol are all commonly prescribed medications to treat which condition?
(A) High blood pressure
(B) High cholesterol
(C) Diabetes
(D) Bacterial infections

88. When collecting a specimen by capillary puncture, what should the MA avoid doing?
(A) Scraping the collection container against the puncture site
(B) Gently squeezing and releasing the finger
(C) Placing the lancet at a 90-degree angle to fingerprint lines
(D) Telling the patient that the puncture may hurt briefly

89. If an MA is assisting with a Pap test, when should she apply fixative to the microscope slides?
(A) Before the provider collects the cells
(B) Immediately after the provider collects the cells
(C) After 5 minutes
(D) After the patient has dressed and left to check out

90. What should be offered to a patient if a provider will be delayed more than 30 minutes?
(A) The chance to reschedule the appointment
(B) A bottle of water or another beverage
(C) A discount on the cost of service
(D) Access to a more comfortable waiting area

91. Services such as anesthesia, surgery, and postoperative care are billed together using ___________ codes.
(A) Unified
(B) Gathered
(C) Joint
(D) Bundled

92. A patient who just received a serious diagnosis starts crying as the MA walks her to check out. Which of the following is the best response from the MA?
(A) "Don't worry. Everything is going to be OK."
(B) "It might be a good idea to get a second opinion."
(C) "This must be so overwhelming. Would you like to sit down somewhere private for a bit?"
(D) "We see patients get through this all the time. We'll make sure you do, too."

93. As he is preparing to place electrodes on a patient's chest for an EKG, an MA notices that the patient has severe acne on his chest. What measure should the MA take?
(A) He should wash the patient's chest with a gentle soap.
(B) He should place the electrodes on the patient's back.
(C) He should wear gloves while conducting the EKG.
(D) He should point at the correct locations and ask the patient to place the electrodes himself.

94. What does administering an intramuscular injection using the Z-track method achieve?
(A) It makes the injection less painful for the patient.
(B) It makes the medication less likely to leak out.
(C) It makes the medication available to the body more quickly.
(D) It puts the medication deeper into the muscle.

Name: ______________________________

95. Which of the following is a contraindication for hormonal forms of birth control?
    (A) History of blood clots
    (B) History of recurring yeast infections
    (C) History of gastric ulcers
    (D) History of high blood pressure

96. What level of asepsis is required for laceration repair?
    (A) Routine asepsis
    (B) Medical asepsis
    (C) Accelerated asepsis
    (D) Surgical asepsis

97. Which are the two main body systems involved in electromyography?
    (A) The nervous system and the circulatory system
    (B) The nervous system and the musculoskeletal system
    (C) The musculoskeletal system and the circulatory system
    (D) The gastrointestinal system and the urinary system

98. What type of business assists medical offices by checking, submitting, and tracking health insurance claims for providers?
    (A) Coding agencies
    (B) Bookkeeping companies
    (C) Clearinghouses
    (D) Payroll managers

99. MAs commonly have these tasks related to specialist referrals:
    (A) Getting preauthorization and making the appointment for the patient
    (B) Giving the patient a list of specialists and documenting which one the patient chooses
    (C) Getting preauthorization and providing the specialist with copies of all of the patient's files
    (D) Making the appointment for the patient and ordering any tests the specialist suggests

100. A patient must follow a low-residue diet for several days. Which of these foods is acceptable on this diet?
    (A) A hamburger without vegetables or condiments
    (B) Chicken breast meat wrapped in a flour tortilla
    (C) Shredded wheat with berries and yogurt
    (D) Salad

101. What is one significant difference between irritable bowel syndrome (IBS) and inflammatory bowel disease (IBD)?
    (A) IBD causes diarrhea and IBS causes constipation.
    (B) Diet changes are helpful for IBD but not for IBS.
    (C) IBS is caused by a problem with bowel function and IBD is caused by physical damage.
    (D) IBS is usually treated with surgery and IBD is treated with medications.

102. Which of these lists venipuncture tubes in the correct order of draw?
    (A) Citrate tube, oxalate tube, EDTA tube
    (B) Oxalate tube, EDTA tube, citrate tube
    (C) EDTA tube, citrate tube, oxalate tube
    (D) Citrate tube, EDTA tube, oxalate tube

103. What anatomical structure should an MA avoid to help prevent gagging during a throat culture?
    (A) The tonsils
    (B) The palate
    (C) The tongue
    (D) The uvula

104. Which of the following should be confirmed during check-in at every patient appointment?
    (A) That the patient still consents to have the provider treat them
    (B) That the patient still has the same insurance
    (C) That the patient understands the office's privacy policies
    (D) Whether the patient has an advance directive

Name: ______________________________

105. An adult patient who does not read may have distant vision tested using a chart that shows
   (A) The letter "E" pointing in different directions
   (B) Shapes or numbers in contrasting colors
   (C) Pictures such as sailboats, stars, and hearts
   (D) Logos from familiar businesses

106. If a patient is always accompanied by another person who does not allow the patient to speak for himself, the MA should document this and report to the provider because this could be a sign of
   (A) Active neglect
   (B) Passive neglect
   (C) Abuse or exploitation
   (D) Entrapment

107. A patient with high blood pressure is seen for chest congestion, general malaise, and a low fever. The provider diagnoses her with bronchitis. What class of medication must be taken with care by a patient with hypertension?
   (A) Antipyretics
   (B) Antitussives
   (C) Decongestants
   (D) Antihistamines

108. Which form of contraception can also prevent or slow the spread of sexually transmitted infections?
   (A) Diaphragm with spermicide
   (B) IUD
   (C) Implanted contraceptives
   (D) Condoms

109. When performing eye irrigation, where should the MA aim the syringe to instill the solution?
   (A) Toward the medial corner of the eye
   (B) Toward the lateral corner of the eye
   (C) Toward the upper eyelid
   (D) Toward the lower eyelid

110. When using a button-activated lancet to perform dermal puncture, how should the MA activate the lancet?
   (A) By pressing the lancet firmly into the patient's skin and then pushing the button
   (B) By placing the lancet against the patient's skin without additional pressure and then pushing the button
   (C) By asking the patient to press the lancet into his own skin depending on his level of comfort and then pushing the button
   (D) By holding the lancet just above the patient's skin and then pushing the button

111. Where does oxygenated blood exit the heart to be pumped to the body?
   (A) Through the superior vena cava
   (B) Through the inferior vena cava
   (C) Through the aorta
   (D) Through the atria

112. A patient with high cholesterol has asked for ideas on nonmeat protein sources to add to his diet. Which of the following lists of foods best meets the patient's needs?
   (A) Cheese, yogurt, and eggs
   (B) Nuts, tofu, and legumes
   (C) Bread, cheese, and cereal
   (D) Salads, seeds, and whole milk dairy products

113. This class of drug may be indicated for cancer patients who are undergoing chemotherapy:
   (A) Antiemetics
   (B) Antihistamines
   (C) Antihyperlipidemic agents
   (D) Anticonvulsants

114. Compared to a patient who has had a broken neck, a patient who has had an injury to the lumbar spine will experience
   (A) No loss of function
   (B) Less loss of function
   (C) About the same loss of function
   (D) More loss of function

115. A patient becomes angry after an MA accidentally bumps his head with a scale's height level during intake. She apologizes but he uses abusive language and then threatens to have her fired. What is the best response by the MA?
(A) "Well, since you're the one being a jerk I don't think that will happen."
(B) "I'd like to see you try."
(C) "I think you have a good point. I'm probably not cut out for this job."
(D) "I'm truly sorry to have hurt you, but please do not use that kind of language in our office."

116. Which of these organs is located entirely within the left upper quadrant of the abdomen?
(A) Stomach
(B) Gallbladder
(C) Liver
(D) Appendix

117. When a patient receives a vaccine, what link in the chain of infection may be broken?
(A) Causative agent
(B) Portal of entry
(C) Mode of transmission
(D) Susceptible host

118. An MA receives a call from a medical office in another city. A patient has moved and his new doctor's office is asking for his records. What must the MA get before sharing the records?
(A) Confirmation that the patient has, in fact, moved
(B) Permission from the provider she works for to share records with the new provider
(C) A signed release from the patient authorizing her to provide the records to the new doctor
(D) Access to an encrypted account for sharing confidential information

119. Testing DTRs involves which of these examination techniques?
(A) Percussion
(B) Auscultation
(C) Palpation
(D) Observation

120. When is it acceptable to use an alcohol-based hand rub rather than soap and water?
(A) When the MA's hands are chapped from washing
(B) When the hands are not visibly soiled
(C) When the MA washed hands within the past 30 minutes
(D) When the patient does not have a diagnosis of *C. difficile*

121. When this condition is not controlled it can lead to heart attack, stroke, reduced circulation, poor wound healing, and kidney and nerve damage:
(A) High blood pressure
(B) Hypothyroidism
(C) Diabetes
(D) Rheumatoid arthritis

122. Professionalism for an MA includes
(A) Wearing a clean and wrinkle-free uniform
(B) Providing informed advice to patients about their conditions
(C) Choosing which waiting patient has the greatest need to see the provider
(D) Being tactful when calling patients to tell them about new diagnoses

123. During a woman's first prenatal visit her pregnancy may be confirmed by testing for the hormone
(A) Progesterone
(B) Antidiuretic hormone
(C) Human growth hormone
(D) Human chorionic gonadotropin

124. A blood test that requires whole blood, such as erythrocyte sedimentation rate, must be collected in a tube that has what kind of additive?
(A) Clot activator
(B) Preservative
(C) Anticoagulant
(D) Separator gel

125. When might a split urine specimen be collected?
(A) When testing for drugs
(B) When testing for pregnancy
(C) When testing ketones
(D) When testing specific gravity

Name: ____________________

126. How is the heart muscle supplied with oxygenated blood?
   (A) It is absorbed through the chambers of the heart.
   (B) It is pumped to the heart muscle through the *venae cavae*.
   (C) It is pumped to the heart muscle through the pulmonary arteries.
   (D) It is pumped to the heart muscle through the coronary arteries.

127. Which body cavity contains the bladder?
   (A) The abdominal cavity
   (B) The pelvic cavity
   (C) The mediastinum
   (D) The orbital cavity

128. What should an MA do before taking a urine specimen from a patient?
   (A) Put on gloves
   (B) Perform a sterile scrub
   (C) Alert the laboratory that a specimen will be delivered
   (D) Ask the patient to wash the outside of the container

129. Which of the following is the best way to ask a patient to confirm his identity?
   (A) "Are you Jade Allen, born 12/9/1972?"
   (B) "Can you state your name and date of birth for me, Ms. Allen?"
   (C) "Can you please state and spell your name and state your date of birth?"
   (D) "Can you state your name and confirm you were born 12/9/1972?"

130. What should a patient be told to avoid for 24 hours before a stress test?
   (A) Exercise
   (B) Caffeine
   (C) Eating and drinking anything other than water
   (D) Taking any kind of medication

131. How long are most blood specimens centrifuged?
   (A) 5–10 minutes
   (B) 10–15 minutes
   (C) 20–30 minutes
   (D) 1 hour

132. A patient who has unstable angina experiences pain
   (A) Only during exercise
   (B) Only at times of intense stress
   (C) When moving from a seated to a standing position
   (D) At rest or without stress

133. When a patient calls to schedule an appointment, the MA needs to know
   (A) Any existing chronic diagnoses
   (B) What medications the patient takes
   (C) Whether the patient has a family history of heart disease
   (D) Whether the patient has been seen at the office before

134. Which of the following must be reported?
   (A) A patient who has a gunshot wound
   (B) A patient who says she cut herself while cooking
   (C) A patient who steps on a rusty nail
   (D) A patient who reports using illegal drugs

135. Confusion is often a symptom of what condition in elderly patients?
   (A) Diabetes
   (B) Urinary tract infection
   (C) Coronary artery disease
   (D) Upper respiratory tract infection

136. *CPOE* stands for
   (A) Computerized physician outpatient education
   (B) Computerized provider order entry
   (C) Computerized preauthorization observation and evaluation
   (D) Computer palpation and observation entry

137. What is one reason to perform venipuncture at an angle no higher than 30 degrees?
   (A) It is more comfortable for the patient.
   (B) It provides more accurate results.
   (C) It reduces the risk of hitting an artery or nerve.
   (D) It is easier for the MA.

138. After donning gloves, an MA notices a small tear in one of them. What should he do?
   (A) Use the glove if the tear is not close to the fingers
   (B) Use the glove if the tear is less than 3 millimeters long
   (C) Use the glove if the patient the MA is working with does not have a bloodborne disease
   (D) Remove and replace the torn glove

139. How can a provider terminate a relationship with an established patient?
   (A) Providers are not permitted to do this; they are obligated to provide care.
   (B) Providers must inform the patient in writing by certified mail and give the patient time to find a new provider.
   (C) Providers must place at least 3 documented phone calls to inform the patient and give the patient time to find a new provider.
   (D) Providers can simply inform their support staff to no longer book appointments with the patient.

140. How is peak flow determined?
   (A) After 3 successful readings are taken, the readings are averaged.
   (B) After 3 successful readings are taken, the highest reading is used.
   (C) After 3 successful readings are taken, the lowest reading is used.
   (D) The patient measures peak flow for a week and the readings are averaged.

141. Which of these is the best site for an insulin injection?
   (A) The deltoid muscle
   (B) The inner forearm
   (C) The back of the upper arm
   (D) The thigh muscle

142. During intake a patient describes back pain he has been having. The MA documents in this way: "Pt. states 'When I bend in any direction it feels like someone is stabbing me on the right side of my lower back.'" Which of the Six Cs of Charting does this note demonstrate best?
   (A) Client's words
   (B) Clarity
   (C) Conciseness
   (D) Completeness

143. How many antiseptic agents are used when preparing a surgical site?
   (A) 1
   (B) 2
   (C) 3
   (D) 4

144. Why should a patient be observed for 20–30 minutes after an allergy injection is administered?
   (A) Because allergy injections often cause dizziness
   (B) Because after 20–30 minutes the MA can report whether the treatment was successful
   (C) Because the injection is most effective if the patient rests right after receiving it
   (D) Because allergy injections can cause anaphylaxis

145. A patient tells the MA, "I have a bad, phlegmy cough and a fever." This is an example of
   (A) Medical history
   (B) Chief complaint
   (C) History of present illness
   (D) Objective information

146. What type of treatment is a patient with a surgically created arteriovenous fistula likely receiving?
   (A) Chemotherapy
   (B) Radiation therapy
   (C) Hemodialysis
   (D) Peritoneal dialysis

Name: ______________________________

147. An MA is placing electrodes for an EKG and sees a pacemaker scar. The patient confirms that he has a pacemaker. What might the MA expect to see on the EKG tracing?
  (A) P waves that go down, rather than up, from the baseline
  (B) Wide, irregular QRS complexes
  (C) Long spaces between the P wave and the R wave
  (D) Spike-like markings

148. Which of these forms of prenatal screening involves the highest degree of risk to the fetus?
  (A) Chorionic villus sampling
  (B) Nuchal translucency test
  (C) Alpha fetoprotein blood test
  (D) Ultrasound

149. Why does atrial fibrillation increase a patient's risk of a stroke?
  (A) Because it causes blood to pool in the brain
  (B) Because pooled blood in the heart may clot and travel to the brain
  (C) Because it increases the risk of a ruptured blood vessel in the brain
  (D) Because it elevates blood pressure

150. Which of the following is true?
  (A) A patient is the owner of their medical record and must be given a complete, free copy upon request.
  (B) A patient is the owner of their medical record but a medical office can charge a reasonable fee for providing the patient with a paper copy.
  (C) The medical office owns a patient's medical record but must provide the patient with a complete, free copy upon request.
  (D) The medical office owns a patient's medical record and can charge a reasonable fee for providing the patient with a paper copy.